Chronic Rhinosinusitis

Guest Editor

WYTSKE J. FOKKENS, MD

IMMUNOLOGY AND ALLERGY CLINICS OF NORTH AMERICA

www.immunology.theclinics.com

Consulting Editor
RAFEUL ALAM, MD, PhD

November 2009 • Volume 29 • Number 4

SAUNDERS an imprint of ELSEVIER, Inc.

W.B. SAUNDERS COMPANY
A Division of Elsevier Inc.

1600 John F. Kennedy Blvd., • Suite 1800 • Philadelphia, PA 19103-2899.

http://www.theclinics.com

IMMUNOLOGY AND ALLERGY CLINICS OF NORTH AMERICA Volume 29, Number 4
November 2009 ISSN 0889–8561, ISBN-13: 978-1-4377-1230-8, ISBN-10: 1-4377-1230-4

Editor: Patrick Manley

Immunology and Allergy Clinics of North America (ISSN 0889–8561) is published quarterly by Elsevier Inc., 360 Park Avenue South, New York, NY 10010-1710. Months of issue are February, May, August, and November. Periodicals postage paid at New York, NY and additional mailing offices. Subscription prices are $254.00 per year for US individuals, $373.00 per year for US institutions, $123.00 per year for US students and residents, $312.00 per year for Canadian individuals, $178.00 per year for Canadian students, $463.00 per year for Canadian institutions, $354.00 per year for international individuals, $463.00 per year for international institutions, and $178.00 per year for international students. To receive student/resident rate, orders must be accompanied by name of affiliated institution, date of term, and the *signature* of program/residency coordinator on institution letterhead. Orders will be billed at individual rate until proof of status is received. Foreign air speed delivery is included in all *Clinics* subscription prices. All prices are subject to change without notice. **POSTMASTER:** Send address changes to *Immunology and Allergy Clinics of North America*, Elsevier Health Sciences Division, Subscription Customer Service, 3251 Riverport Lane, Maryland Heights, MO 63043. **Customer Service: 1-800-654-2452 (U.S. and Canada); 314-447-8871 (outside U.S. and Canada). Fax: 314-447-8029. E-mail: journalscustomerservice-usa@elsevier.com (for print support); journalsonlinesupport-usa@elsevier.com (for online support).**

Reprints. For copies of 100 or more, of articles in this publication, please contact the Commercial Reprints Department, Elsevier Inc., 360 Park Avenue South, New York, New York 10010-1710. Tel. (212) 633-3812, Fax: (212) 462-1935, e-mail: reprints@elsevier.com.

Immunology and Allergy Clinics of North America is covered in MEDLINE/PubMed (Index Medicus), Current Contents/Life Sciences, Science Citation Index, ISI/BIOMED, Chemical Abstracts, and EMBASE/Excerpta Medica.

Printed and bound by CPI Group (UK) Ltd, Croydon, CR0 4YY
Transferred to Digital Print 2011

Contributors

CONSULTING EDITOR

RAFEUL ALAM, MD, PhD
Veda and Chauncey Ritter Chair in Immunology, Professor, and Director, Division of Immunology and Allergy, National Jewish Health; and University of Colorado Health Sciences Center, Denver, Colorado

GUEST EDITOR

WYTSKE J. FOKKENS, MD, PhD
Professor and Chair, Department of Otorhinolaryngology, Academic Medical Center, Amsterdam, The Netherlands

AUTHORS

ISAM ALOBID, MD, PhD
Unitat de Rinologia & Clínica de l'Olfacte, Department of Otorhinolaryngology, Hospital Clínic, Catalonia, Spain

MARCELO B. ANTUNES, MD
Instructor, Department of Otorhinolaryngology–Head and Neck Surgery, University of Pennsylvania School of Medicine, Philadelphia, Pennsylvania

NEIL BHATTACHARYYA, MD
Associate Professor of Otology and Laryngology, Division of Otolaryngology, Department of Otology, Rhinology, and Laryngology, Brigham and Women's Hospital, Harvard Medical School, Boston, Massachusetts

NOAM A. COHEN, MD, PhD
Assistant Professor, Department of Otorhinolaryngology–Head and Neck Surgery, University of Pennsylvania School of Medicine, Philadelphia, Pennsylvania

MARTIN Y. DESROSIERS, MD
Associate Professor, Department of Otolaryngology, Hôpital Hôtel-Dieu, Université de Montréal; and Department of Otolaryngology, McGill University, Montreal, Quebec, Canada

FENNA EBBENS, MD, PhD
Department of Otorhinolaryngology, Academic Medical Center, Amsterdam, The Netherlands

BERRYLIN J. FERGUSON, MD
Associate Professor and Director, Division of Sinonasal Disorders and Allergy, Department of Otolaryngology, University of Pittsburgh School of Medicine, University of Pittsburgh Medical Center, Pittsburgh, Pennsylvania

WYTSKE J. FOKKENS, MD, PhD
Professor and Chair, Department of Otorhinolaryngology, Academic Medical Center, Amsterdam, The Netherlands

DAVID A. GUDIS, MD
Instructor, Department of Otorhinolaryngology–Head and Neck Surgery, University of Pennsylvania School of Medicine, Philadelphia, Pennsylvania

RICHARD J. HARVEY, MD
Department of Otolaryngology, Skull Base Surgery, St. Vincent's, Hospital, Darlinghurst, Sydney, Australia

PETER W. HELLINGS, MD, PhD
Professor and Doctor, Department of Otorhinolaryngology, Head, and Neck Surgery, University Hospitals Leuven, Catholic University of Leuven, Leuven, Belgium

GREET HENS, MD, PhD
Doctor, Department of Otorhinolaryngology, Head, and Neck Surgery, University Hospitals Leuven, Catholic University of Leuven, Leuven, Belgium

SHAUN J. KILTY, MD
Assistant Professor, The Department of Otolaryngology—Head and Neck Surgery, University of Ottawa, Ottawa, Ontario, Canada

L. KLIMEK, MD, PhD
Professor, Center for Rhinology and Allergy, Wiesbaden, Germany

VALERIE J. LUND, MD
Professor of Rhinology and Honorary Consultant ENT Surgeon, Rhinology Research Unit, The Royal National Throat, Nose and Ear Hospital, London, United Kingdom

JOAQUIM MULLOL, MD, PhD
Unitat de Rinologia & Clínica de l'Olfacte, Department of Otorhinolaryngology, Hospital Clínic; and Clinical and Experimental Respiratory Immunoallergy, Institut d'Investigacions Biomédiques August Pi i Sunyer, Catalonia, Spain

ANDRÉS OBANDO, MD
Unitat de Rinologia & Clínica de l'Olfacte, Department of Otorhinolaryngology, Hospital Clínic, Catalonia, Spain

BRADLEY A. OTTO, MD
Division of Sinus and Allergy, Department of Otolaryngology-Head and Neck Surgery, The Ohio State University, Columbus, Ohio

HARSHITA PANT, BMBS, PhD
Division of Sinonasal Disorders and Allergy, Department of Otolaryngology, University of Pittsburgh School of Medicine, University of Pittsburgh Medical Center, Pittsburgh, Pennsylvania

O. PFAAR, MD
Center for Rhinology and Allergy, Wiesbaden, Germany

LAURA PUJOLS, PhD
Clinical and Experimental Respiratory Immunoallergy, Institut d'Investigacions
Biomèdiques August Pi i Sunyer, Catalonia, Spain

SUSANNE REINARTZ, MD
Department of Otorhinolaryngology, Academic Medical Center, Amsterdam, The
Netherlands

NINA L. SHAPIRO, MD
Associate Professor of Surgery, Division of Head and Neck Surgery, David Geffen School
of Medicine at University of California Los Angeles, Los Angeles, California

CORNELIS M. VAN DRUNEN, PhD
Head ENT Research Laboratory, Department of Otorhinolaryngology, Academic Medical
Center, Amsterdam, The Netherlands

BEN D. WALLWORK, MD, PhD
Department of Otolaryngology, Princess Alexandra Hospital, Brisbane, Queensland,
Australia

JOCHEM WIGMAN, MD
Department of Otorhinolaryngology, Academic Medical Center, Amsterdam, The
Netherlands

ARTHUR W. WU, MD
Division of Head and Neck Surgery, David Geffen School of Medicine at University
of California Los Angeles, Los Angeles, California

Contents

and oral corticosteroids, constitutes its first line of therapy. Long-term treatment with corticosteroid nasal spray reduces inflammation and nasal polyp size, and improves nasal symptoms such as nasal blockage, rhinorrea, and the loss of smell. Corticosteroid intranasal drops may be used when intranasal spray fails to demonstrate efficacy. Short courses of oral steroids are recommended in severe chronic rhinosinusitis with nasal polyps or when a rapid symptomatic improvement is needed. Endoscopic sinus surgery is only recommended when the medical treatment fails. Intranasal corticosteroids should be continued postoperatively. When using intranasal corticosteroids, care should be taken in selected populations such as children, pregnant women, and elderly patients; especially in those patients with comorbid conditions such as asthma, in which the overall steroid intake can be high due to the administration of both intranasal and inhaled corticosteroids.

Intolerance to acetylsalicylic acid and to other nonsteroidal anti-inflammatory drugs was first described in 1922. The clinical picture reveals a classic triad of symptoms: aspirin-induced bronchial asthma, aspirin sensitivity, and chronic rhinosinusitis with nasal polyps. In many cases, nasal polyps reveal as the first symptom of ASA sensitivity, indicating that the upper airways are predominantly involved in the pathogenetic process. The emphasis of this article is on the upper airways of ASA-intolerant patients. Imbalance of the eicosanoids leukotrienes and prostaglandins might be the pathophysiologic key to the disease. The patient's history and challenge tests with lysine-aspirin are the diagnostic tools of choice. Apart from surgical or pharmacologic therapy, ASA-desensitization therapy is the treatment of choice. Various desensitization protocols and routes of administration are discussed.

Fungal spores, due to their ubiquitous nature, are continuously inhaled and deposited on the airway mucosa. This article focuses on the potential role of fungi in chronic rhinosinusitis (CRS). Five forms of fungal disease affecting the nose and paranasal sinuses have been recognized: (1) acute invasive fungal rhinosinusitis (including rhinocerebral mucormycosis), (2) chronic invasive fungal rhinosinusitis, (3) granulomatous invasive fungal rhinosinusitis, (4) fungal ball (mycetoma), and (5) noninvasive (allergic) fungal rhinosinusitis. There are several potential deficits in the innate and potentially also acquired immunity of CRS patients that might reduce or change their ability to react to fungi. There are not many arguments to suggest a causative role for fungi in CRS with or without nasal polyps. However, due to the intrinsic or induced change in immunity of CRS patients, fungi might have a disease-modifying role.

The anti-inflammatory effects of macrolides are significant. The clinical impact on diffuse panbronchiolitis (DPB) has improved 10-year survival from 12% to more than 90% for these patients. The immunomodulatory activity of macrolides has been a source of mechanistic research as well as clinical research in non-DPB inflammatory airway disease. Suppression of neutrophilic inflammation of the airways has been demonstrated as the most robust immunomodulatory response from 14- and 15-membered ring macrolides. The inhibition of transcription factors, mainly nuclear factor-kB and activator protein 1, from alterations in intracellular cell signaling drives this mechanism. The suppression of interleukin-8 to a range of endogenous and exogenous challenges characterizes the alterations to cytokine production. The inflammatory mechanisms of chronic rhinosinusitis (CRS) have been a major non-DPB focus. Macrolides have been trialed in more than 14 prospective trials and are the focus of numerous research projects. Evidence for a strong clinical effect in CRS is mounting, but results may be tempered by researchers' inability to characterize the disease process. Eosinophilic dominated CRS is unlikely to respond, based on current research understanding and data from clinical trials. This article discusses the current concepts of macrolides and their application in the management of CRS.

Pediatric chronic rhinosinusitis, a common problem, has been found to have a severe impact on the quality of life. As in the case with adult chronic rhinosinusitis, pediatric chronic rhinosinusitis is difficult to treat, with resultant frequent recurrences and failures. Controversy has existed in the treatment of chronic rhinosinusitis in children, mirroring the controversy over the exact etiology of this disorder. Chronic rhinosinusitis may indeed be a group of diseases with similar presenting features. This article attempts to delineate treatment options that are both safe and effective for pediatric chronic rhinosinusitis.

This article examines the modalities in the treatment of chronic rhinosinusitis (CRS). A correct diagnosis is the first requirement in the successful management of CRS. CRS-directed therapy might fail if the actual cause of symptoms is nonsinogenic. Nasal endoscopy and sinus computed tomography are the primary modalities used in the diagnosis of sinusitis. Allergy and gastroesophageal reflux, may not directly cause sinusitis, but they frequently mimic the symptoms of sinusitis. Therapy can include avoidance of allergens and desensitization in the former and antireflux therapy in the latter. Underlying systemic causes of refractory sinusitis include immunodeficiency and systemic granulomatous and eosinophilic syndromes. Correct diagnosis is essential to directed therapy. Patients with aspirin exacerbated respiratory disease may benefit from aspirin desensitization. Optimization of mucociliary clearance can be augmented with nasal lavage and mucolytics. Additional nonsteroidal antiinflammatory modalities include use of the leukotriene modulators, montelukast and zileuton. Patients with elevated IgE may benefit from omalizumab (anti-IgE); however, cost constraints restrict use to those patients who have severe asthma. This article also includes management strategies beyond the usual antibiotics, steroids, and sinus surgery. Once immunodeficiency and confounding local mimics of sinusitis are addressed, additional interventions should be tried separately initially to assess the individual patient's response to therapy.

The interaction between upper and lower airway disease has been recognized for centuries, with recent studies showing a direct link between upper and airway inflammation in allergic patients. The mechanisms underlying the interaction between nasal and bronchial inflammation have primarily been studied in allergic disease, showing systemic immune activation after allergen inhalation, induction of inflammation at a distance, and a negative impact of nasal inflammation on bronchial homeostasis. Therefore, allergic rhinitis and asthma are considered part of the global airway allergy syndrome. Besides allergy, other inflammatory conditions such as the common cold, acute rhinosinusitis, and chronic rhinosinusitis are associated with lower airway disease. Chronic sinus disease with or without nasal polyps are frequently found in patients with asthma and chronic obstructive pulmonary disease with improvement of bronchial symptoms and respiratory function by adequate medical and surgical therapy for rhinosinusitis. The resolution of sinonasal inflammation and hence sinonasal functions by medical or surgical treatment is considered responsible for the beneficial effect of treatment on bronchial disease. This article aims at providing a comprehensive overview of the current knowledge on the interaction between common cold, acute and chronic rhinosinusitis, and lower airway biology.

THE CLINICS ARE NOW AVAILABLE ONLINE!

Access your subscription at:
www.theclinics.com

Foreword: Chronic Sinusitis

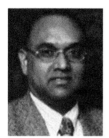

Rafeul Alam, MD, PhD
Consulting Editor

Most medical textbooks do not have a chapter on chronic sinusitis. Yet this is a debilitating disease for many patients. It is one of the most poorly researched human illnesses. As a result, understanding of this illness is superficial, and the management approach is inadequate and not satisfactory to many patients. There are many issues that are unresolved. Chronic sinusitis is certainly a heterogeneous disease but how many different subtypes are there? What is the role of allergy? Why do so many patients have a negative skin test yet manifest T_H2 inflammation that is rich in eosinophils? What is the role of eocosanoids in polypoid growth in nonsteroidal anti-inflammatory drug (NSAID)-intolerant versus NSAID-tolerant patients? Does IgE participate in the pathogenesis? What is the role of infection? What about fungi?

A major hindrance to advancing knowledge in chronic sinusitis is the difficulty in accessing sinus tissue or other biologic samples for research. Unless this problem is overcome, the knowledge about chronic sinusitis will remain inadequate. The immune system plays an important role in this disease but it has not been aggressively investigated compared to asthma or allergic rhinitis. Sinus CT is helpful but the readout is subjective and a quantitative approach is needed. Its high cost is a limiting factor, especially for monitoring treatment efficacy. A biomarker for the disease would be useful. Finally, some treatment approaches to chronic sinusitis have been a matter of controversy. There a few well-controlled studies. The patient populations for these studies are not well characterized, making interpretation of the results difficult.

Dr. Wytske Fokkens and colleagues have been at the forefront of this challenging topic. She has invited an international group of experts to provide updates on the many aspects of chronic sinusitis. This is an important addition to *Immunology and Allergy Clinics of North America*.

Rafeul Alam, MD, PhD
Division of Allergy and Immunology
National Jewish Health and University of Colorado Denver Health Sciences Center
1400 Jackson Street, Denver, CO 80206, USA

E-mail address:
alamr@njc.org

Immunol Allergy Clin N Am 29 (2009) xiii
doi:10.1016/j.iac.2009.08.003   immunology.theclinics.com

Preface

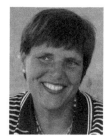

Wytske J. Fokkens, MD, PhD
Guest Editor

Rhinosinusitis is a significant and increasing health problem that results in a large financial burden on society. Rhinitis and sinusitis usually coexist and are concurrent in most individuals; thus, the correct terminology is now rhinosinusitis. Rhinosinusitis (including nasal polyps) is defined as inflammation of the nose and the paranasal sinuses characterized by nasal blockage, nasal discharge (anterior/posterior nasal drip), facial pain/pressure, or reduction or loss of smell, and endoscopic signs of polyps or mucopurulent discharge primarily from middle meatus, edema/mucosal obstruction primarily in middle meatus, or CT changes showing mucosal changes within the ostiomeatal complex or sinuses.

The past decade has made it clear that chronic rhinosinusitis (CRS) is not an infectious disease but that the pathophysiology is multifactorial. The exact pathophysiology is far from clear but in recent years different investigators have pointed to the small role of anatomic abnormalities and the large role of inflammation. Different causes of inflammation have been explored, such as allergy, inflammatory response to fungal or bacterial elements, disorders in the immunity of patients, aspirin, and the role of biofilms. In accordance with the limited role of blocked ostia as the primary cause of the disease, the focus of treatment has changed from sinus surgery to medical treatment of inflammation, leaving surgery as the last resort.

In this issue of the *Immunology and Allergy Clinics of North America*, authorities in the field give their views on current understanding of the causes of CRS and its management. CRS is increasingly thought to be inflammatory. Kees van Drunen focuses on current understanding of the cellular makeup of the inflammatory influx in CRS in relationship to the different expression forms of CRS. Traditionally, research focused on the role of eosinophils in the pathogenic mechanisms but recently more attention has been given to neutrophils and to different T-lymphocyte subtypes. His article summarizes current understanding and discusses opportunities and potential pitfalls related to inflammation-related research. Not only influx of inflammatory cells but also the role of more residential cells of the nasal mucosa is of increased interest. Noam Cohen and colleagues focus on the important role of the mucociliary clearance

doi:10.1016/j.iac.2009.08.002
0889-8561/09/$ – see front matter © 2009 Elsevier Inc. All rights reserved.
immunology.theclinics.com

in the primary innate defense of the nasal and sinus mucosa and how the mucociliary components function and their impairment may contribute to the development and progression of CRS.

Although it is increasingly clear that bacterial infection in itself is not the cause of CRS, infection in the form of biofilm may have an important role in the maintenance of the recalcitrant inflammation. Shaun Kilty and Martin Desrosiers put forward that biofilm disease has a central role in dictating the clinical manifestations of the disease while also accounting for its recurrent nature. This suggests that the development of rapid clinical tests that facilitate diagnosis are a prerequisite for effective eradication or control of the biofilm-forming bacteria by the production of efficacious and safe topical treatment.

There several potential deficits in the innate and potentially acquired immunity of CRS patients that might reduce or change their ability to react to fungi. Although persuasively promoted in the past decade, there are not many arguments to suggest a causative role for fungi in CRS with or without nasal polyps. Due to the intrinsic or induced change in immunity of CRS patients, however, fungi may have a disease-modifying role. The inability to reduce symptoms and signs of CRS inflammation by antifungal treatment, however, moderates enthusiasm for putting a great deal of effort into further unraveling this role.

Lutger Klimek and Oliver Pfaar focus on the potential role of aspirin intolerance and the potential of aspirin desensitization to alter the course of the disease. They maintain that desensitization reduces the growth and recurrence rate of nasal polyps in aspirin-sensitive patients over a longer time period, offering further suggestions for treating patients with CRS with nasal polyps.

For many years corticosteroids have been the workhorse of CRS treatment. Joachim Mullol and colleagues summarize the mechanism of action, pharmacology, and clinical relevance of corticosteroids in the treatment of CRS with and without nasal polyps.

Richard Harvey and Valerie Lund discuss the rationale and evidence for use of macrolides in the treatment of CRS. They argue that the suppression of neutrophilic inflammation of the airways has been demonstrated, as the most robust immunomodulatory response of macrolides and eosinophilic-dominated CRS is unlikely to respond based on current research understanding and data from clinical trials. Larger clinical trials are needed, preferably combined with studies of the inflammatory process in the same patients to further elucidate the role of macrolides in CRS.

In some patients, CRS can be extremely recalcitrant, driving doctors and patients to despair. Berrylin Ferguson and colleagues offer suggestions for differential diagnosis and treatment options when intranasal and systemic antibiotics, corticosteroids, and endoscopic sinus surgery fail. They propose several additional interventions that can be tried in patients with recalcitrant CRS, although evidence of their efficacy (in the total CRS population) is usually lacking. They emphasize the importance of using these interventions initially separately, to assess individual patient response to therapy.

As emphasized by various investigators in this issue, not all patients with CRS are the same. This is especially true for children with CRS. Neil Bhattacharyya and colleagues emphasize that in children, CRS is a common problem that has a severe impact on quality of life. They reason that the controversy that exists in the management of CRS in children mirrors the controversy in adults. Even more than in adults, however, surgical intervention should only be considered for children when "maximal medical therapy" fails.

Finally, Peter Hellings and Greet Hens highlight the importance of the global airway concept in CRS. They propose that the full appreciation of involvement of upper and lower airway disease in one patient can only be executed in a multidisciplinary clinical setting, involving doctors able to examine and interpret clinical abnormalities of upper and lower airways.

Knowledge of the pathophysiology and management of CRS has increased enormously in the past decade. As much as has been learned, however, we are still often blissfully ignorant. I hope this issue will stimulate thoughts, discussions, and research for the benefit of patients.

To be conscience that you are ignorant is a great step to knowledge.
-Benjamin Disraeli (1804–1881).

Wytske J. Fokkens, MD, PhD
Department of Otorhinolaryngology
Academic Medical Center
Amsterdam
The Netherlands

E-mail address:
w.j.fokkens@amc.nl

Inflammation in Chronic Rhinosinusitis and Nasal Polyposis

Cornelis M. van Drunen, PhD*, Susanne Reinartz, MD,
Jochem Wigman, MD, Wytske J. Fokkens, MD, PhD

KEYWORDS

- Chronic rhinosinusitis • Nasal polyposis • Inflammation
- Eosinophils • Neutrophils • Immune regulation

All definitions of chronic rhinosinusitis (CRS) seem to agree on one aspect of the disease: that it involves inflammation. Unfortunately, how united the definitions are on inflammation, so varied the symptoms that develop from this inflammation when patients have to be considered to suffer from CRS. Despite the variety of symptoms, guidelines on CRS classify all sinus diseases as belonging to a single group, albeit that for clinical and basic research purposes the disease can be differentiated into groups depending on the presence or absence of nasal polyps.[1–4] Given the limited medical and surgical treatment options, a single collective is perhaps understandable, but in the long run probably not desirable.

This article focuses on current understanding of the cellular makeup of the inflammatory influx in CRS in relation to the different expression forms of CRS. The first part highlights an ongoing discussion about the role of eosinophils in the pathogenesis of CRS and offsets their presence to neutrophils. This distinction has become relevant in the concept of 2 types of CRS that could be characterized by either eosinophils or neutrophils. The second part focuses on a relatively new aspect, the role of dendritic cells and T lymphocytes in the pathogenesis of CRS. Special interest has recently been given to different subtypes of immune responses (Th1 versus Th2), and a new subtype of T lymphocytes (Th17) that is characterized by the production of interleukin (IL)-17. The final part again steps away from the detailed description of the cellular influx, and discusses specific issues that are important for the interpretation of all the cellular data currently available in the literature.

EOSINOPHILS VERSUS NEUTROPHILS

Probably the most evident misunderstanding in the chronic rhinosinusitis field is that CRS is a pure eosinophilic disease. When the group of CRS patients is considered as

Department of Otorhinolaryngology, Academic Medical Center, Room L3-104-2, PO box 22700, 1100 DE Amsterdam, The Netherlands
* Corresponding author.
E-mail address: c.m.vandrunen@amc.uva.nl (C.M. van Drunen).

Immunol Allergy Clin N Am 29 (2009) 621–629
doi:10.1016/j.iac.2009.07.003
0889-8561/09/$ – see front matter © 2009 Elsevier Inc. All rights reserved.

a whole it is clear that, despite CRS patients displaying different levels of eosinophils, the median values of CRS patients is higher than those of control groups.[5-7] This fact might have triggered the idea that eosinophilia would be present in all individuals, and might also have triggered lines of research that would substantiate the role of the eosinophilia, by focusing solely on related markers (RANTES, Eotaxin, IL-5, eosinophil cationic protein).[8-11] The importance of eosinophils was further strengthened by the introduction of the fungal hypothesis as the sole cause of CRS. In this hypothesis, toxic mediators secreted by eosinophils play an essential role in the elimination of the fungi infection and, as an unwanted side effect, in local tissue destruction and CRS-related symptoms.[12,13] However, the latter hypothesis was dealt a blow when placebo-controlled studies could not show any relevant effectiveness of an antifungal treatment in the alleviation of CRS symptoms or on relevant mediators.[14-17] The former counter-argument that not all CRS patients have eosinophilia is more complex, as the activation state of eosinophils should also be considered, and this cannot be deduced from eosinophil numbers only.[12,18]

Stronger arguments that eosinophils are not the end-all of CRS pathogenesis comes from several directions. Polyps found associated with cystic fibrosis[19,20] and polyps found in the Asian population[21] display hardly any eosinophilia, but are in contrast relatively neutrophilic. Both cystic fibrosis and Asian polyps are indistinguishable macroscopically from regular CRS polyps, showing that at least eosinophilia is not required for polyp formation. This finding is also suggested indirectly by the results of a new treatment option for CRS using anti–IL-5 antibodies.[22] This method is most effective in individuals with increased levels of IL-5, suggestive of an alternative pathogenesis mechanism that is independent of IL-5 and, as a potential consequence, eosinophilia. Upregulation of IL-8, a neutrophil chemokine, has been reported too, but has never been a main focus of research.[23-25] The authors recently were able to independently corroborate these observations at the protein level, showing tissue levels of IL-8 to be more than 5-fold higher in nasal polyps than turbinates from healthy controls.[26]

In a sense the discovery of neutrophils in CRS seems to mirror their discovery in asthma. Whereas asthma was once considered a purely eosinophilic disease, it is now clear that neutrophils are prevalent in difficult-to-treat, nonallergic asthma. For cystic fibrosis polyps this parallel could hold true as they are neutrophilic and, due to the high recurrence levels, should be considered difficult to treat. However, whether the same would hold true for the Asian polyps is not clear.

DENDRITIC CELLS AND T LYMPHOCYTES

In a classic view on the regulation of immune responses, peripheral dendritic cells survey local airway mucosa for potential threats. When such threats have breached the physical epithelial barrier, direct uptake of the pathogen or indirect uptake of an infected tissue cell leads to the initiation of the appropriate immune response. Essential in this process is that the locally activated dendritic cells travel to the corresponding draining lymph node, where they activate naïve T lymphocytes. In the case of a bacterial or viral infection this would result in the formation of the T helper 1 (Th1) subtype; in the case of a parasitic infection this would result in the activation of the T helper 2 (Th2) subtype. These responses are not the only ones possible. In addition to the classic Th1 or Th2 response, a Th17 or T-regulatory response has been identified, with even more responses suspected to exist.[27]

In this light it would seem easy to conceive a role for dendritic cells found in CRS or nasal polyposis (NP) in the initiation or control of a local immune reaction.

However, this idea might not be so straightforward. First there is the issue of the missing pathogen. The pathogenesis of CRS or NP currently remains largely unknown.[1–3] No pathogens have been found that could act as the disease trigger although a bacterial, viral, or fungal source has been hypothesized. Even a local autoimmune reaction cannot be discarded, although also here, the offending target remains elusive. Second, dendritic cells are not only active in the initiation or regulation of an immune response but also in the effector phase of the immune response. When dendritic cells are experimentally removed from a mouse that is already sensitized for ovalbumin, no allergic inflammation reaction can be elicited after ovalbumin exposure.[28] Even when one assumes that local dendritic cells are involved in the regulation of an immune response, the situation remains complex. Given the described comorbidity between allergy and asthma on one hand and CRS/NP on the other hand, most research has focused on local Th2 versus Th1 responses, whereas hardly any data are available on local Th17 or T-regulatory responses.

Similar considerations affect thoughts on the role of local T lymphocytes. In the case of local CD8 lymphocytes, these might well be the cytotoxic T cells fighting a local pathogen or targeting a local autoantigen. In the case of local CD4 lymphocytes, these might be any of the different "helper" cells (Th1, Th2, Th17, or T-regulatory). To make the issue even more complex, within the CD8 family of T lymphocytes a regulatory phenotype has also been identified.[29]

As well as these general considerations affecting potential roles for local dendritic cells or T lymphocytes, there is the issue of a wide variety of comorbidities (allergy, asthma, cystic fibrosis) that are associated with CRS or NP.[1–3] This issue has 2 important consequences related to dendritic cells or T lymphocytes. First, if simple CRS (without comorbidities) would be a different disease modality than CRS with any of the comorbidities, the specific role of dendritic cells or T lymphocytes in the regulation or effector phase of these diseases might well be different. Second, when one would consider allergy and asthma as epiphenomena of CRS or NP, the allergic background of the patient would affect the dendritic cell or T-lymphocyte profiles. This assessment could potentially mask an intrinsic CRS profile of these cells. The dendritic cell or T-lymphocyte profiles can also be affected by the bacterium *Staphylococcus aureus*. Although *S. aureus* should not be considered as a comorbidity of CRS or NP, a substantial group of patients do carry this bacterium in the local tissue. Through its superantigens and allergens *S. aureus* can select for certain dendritic cell HLA- or T-cell receptor (TCR) subtypes that may or may not be directly linked to the disease pathogenesis.[30,31] Finally, the consequences of systemic versus local disease should be considered. Many of the immunologic considerations on CRS/NP stem from a systemic point of view with, for instance, skin prick testing or serology as primary outcome measures of the allergic status. Given that nasal polyps can contain tertiary lymphatic follicles,[32,33] one cannot be sure that the systemic data will correctly describe local tissue events.

No comparison data on dendritic cell subsets are available for CRS. A recent study by Rampey and colleagues[34] investigated the expression of 2 dendritic cell markers, DC-LAMP (CD208) and DC-SIGN (CD209). Other than that cells with these markers were present, no other conclusions could be drawn due to the very small number of patients in this study. A study by Haas and colleagues[35] focused on the then best known dendritic cell, the Langerhans cell. Using CD1a as a marker (that unfortunately can also be found on some macrophages), they showed not only their presence but also that a substantial part of these Langerhans cells carried IgE on their cell surface via the FcεRI.

The most detailed analysis on the phenotypes of T lymphocytes in NP has been performed by Sánchez-Segura and colleagues.[36] Using fluorescence-activated cell sorting (FACS) analysis for multiple markers on cells released from nasal polyp samples, they established that most of the T lymphocytes are activated memory T cells that display a mixed Th1/Th2 phenotype. A strong point of this study is that the patient population (18 subjects in total) is rather homogeneous. Only 2 individuals had established concomitant allergic rhinitis, and one individual had aspirin sensitivity. Furthermore, before surgery the patients had refrained from using steroids for at least 2 months.

Close to 85% of all mononuclear cells in the polyps are CD3+CD45+ T cells, with minor fractions CD19+ B cells or CD56+ NK cells. Nearly of these T cells (87%) express the $\alpha\beta$ TCR with only a minor fraction expressing the $\gamma\delta$ TCR. The activation marker CD69 is relatively highly expressed (77%) whereas CD25 (IL-2 receptor), in contrast, is expressed at a low level (5%). This pattern is very different from the expression pattern of these markers on T cells isolated from the blood of the same patients. In blood, hardly any CD69 can be detected (5%) whereas approximately 25% of the cells express CD25. Although the T lymphocytes from the nasal polyps express high levels of CD45RO and low levels of the adhesion molecule CD62L that would identify these cells as memory T cells, the high level of CD69 is unexpected. Indeed memory cells isolated from the blood do not display this high level of CD69 expression. However, memory T cells with identical marker expression have been observed under other chronic inflammatory conditions like those found in rheumatoid arthritis.[37] Such discrepancies in marker expression between T lymphocytes isolated from the polyp tissue and blood was also observed for CD54, CD62L, CD103, and CD95, suggestive of local processes that affect the phenotype of T lymphocytes. The next important observation from the Sánchez-Segura group is that despite high levels of the Fas death receptor CD95, ligation of the receptor with Fas ligand does not induce apoptosis. This resistance to apoptosis could be a contributing factor to the persistence of inflammation in NP. However, it should be noted that the patients in this (and many other) studies did not respond to steroid treatment, which could mean that these observations are specific for this patient group only and not for NP per se.

To further characterize the T lymphocytes found in nasal polyps, spontaneous or induced (anti-CD3 plus anti-CD28) expression of secreted IL-2, IL-4, IL-5, and interferon (IFN)-γ was investigated. Expression of IL-5 and IFN-γ could be detected only when a mixed Th1/Th2 response was deduced. No data were available to show whether individual T cells secrete both IL-5 and IFN-γ or that 2 sets of T cells exist that each express IL-5 or IFN-γ. Moreover, the absence of IL-4 expression and the missing data on IL-17 (Th17) or IL-10/transforming growth factor (TGF)-β (T-regulatory) makes a firm conclusion on the type of immune response in nasal polyps premature. An independent approach to studying the Th1 or Th2 response was used by Elhini and colleagues[38] through the investigation of chemokine receptors in mucosal biopsies. Expression of CCR5 and CXCR3 is typically found on Th1 cells, whereas CCR4 and CCR8 are mostly found on Th2 cells.[39] However, several differences in the study group prevent the use of these data to confirm or refine the data from Sánchez-Segura's group. Not only did these patients have only CRS and the specimens taken from the mucosa of the ethmoidal sinuses, but the direct comparison in this study was between atopic and nonatopic individuals. Despite these limitations the data did show a positive correlation ($r = +0.9$) between total IgE and CCR4 and a negative correlation ($r = -0.8$) between total IgE and CCR5. This result highlights that cellular phenotypes may strongly depend on existing comorbidities. This same issue may play a role in the observations of Bernstein and colleagues,[40] whereby FACS analysis on polyposis T cells was able to show not only intracellular IL-5 and IFN-γ expression but also IL-2 and IL-4 expression. It is recommended that expression of these cytokines was evaluated for CD4 and CD8 T lymphocytes independently. This point is important, as expression of cytokines differs between these T-cell subtypes and different ratios between CD4 and CD8 T lymphocytes could exist between the different comorbidities. The investigators tried to stratify their data for atopy and aspirin intolerance separately, but the 13 patients in this study were insufficient to stratify for both comorbidities together. This limitation makes the study somewhat underpowered, so that the investigators' conclusion that no differences in expression were evident between the different subgroups remains to be proven.

The research focus recently has shifted toward other T-cell subtypes with a focus on regulatory T cells and the newly discovered Th17 subtype. Van Bruane and colleagues detected differences in T-lymphocyte subtype-specific transcription factors between healthy controls and CRS with polyps or without polyps.[41] In CRS/NP, FOXp3 (T-regulatory cells, activated T cells?) and TGF-β1 (T-regulatory cells, remodeling?) were expressed at a lower level than in controls, whereas T-bet (Th1) and GATA-3 (Th2) were expressed at a higher level. In CRS none of these proteins were affected, but showed a higher level of TGF-β1 (T-regulatory cells, remodeling?) and IFN-γ (Th1?). The interpretation of the data is still difficult, as FOXp3 in man is also expressed by activated T cells, TGF-β1 can be seen as an immune suppressive agent or as a key tissue remodeling factor, and IFN-γ would be both Th1- and antiviral-specific. A potential role of the Th17 subtype is still unclear. Whereas some investigators report increased levels of IL-17 in NP,[42] others were not able to reproduce these data.[41] The latter group, however, did show a Th17 skewed profile in Asian polyps.

INFLAMMATION, COMORBIDITIES, AND STRUCTURAL ASPECTS IN CHRONIC RHINOSINUSITIS

When studying a disease association it is important that the disease is well defined, that all patients suffer from the same disease, and that this group of patients is compared with an appropriate set of controls. Throughout the previous sections, examples of potential caveats have been mentioned and here these are reviewed in a broader context.

First, consider CRS as a single disease. Here one is confronted with the difficulty of defining CRS.[1–4] A wide spectrum of diseases (including vasculitis, Wegener disease, anatomic deviations, and so forth) is described that can underlie CRS, but fortunately most studies will exclude these patients in the analysis of CRS *proper*. The same would hold true for CRS and NP found to be associated with cystic fibrosis or with aspirin intolerance. Although macroscopically difficult to tell apart from NP *proper*, it has been widely recognized that these expressions of CRS could be based on distinctive pathogenic mechanisms. This exclusion leaves a "unique" group of patients for which it is still a struggle to understand whether these are indeed a single group or not. In this group of patients one might encounter a broad range of different inflammatory cells, with some individuals having hardly any inflammatory cells of a given type whereas other individuals may have many of this cell type. This broad range is the reason why data on cellular influxes should be presented as medians and interquartile ranges rather than as average cell numbers or means, as these are too susceptible to a few outliers. With broad ranges of different cell types, it will come as no surprise that one begins to think of potential subtypes of CRS or NP within the previously described "unique" group of patients. The clearest example seems to be the division between "eosinophilic" and "neutrophilic". In addition to the plain observation that some individuals do have more eosinophils whereas others have more neutrophils, several other observations make this distinction reasonable. Polyps found to be associated with cystic fibrosis, whereby one comes to accept a different pathophysiological disease mechanism, are dominated by a neutrophilic influx, with only low numbers of eosinophils. Cystic fibrosis polyps do have increased levels of IL-5, severing the seemingly unbreakable link between IL-5 and eosinophils. Furthermore, nasal polyps found in the Asian population, despite being macroscopically indistinguishable from their Caucasian counterparts, are also mostly neutrophilic. Given the potential existence of 2 subtypes of NP, it remains to be seen whether this is the result of a distinct pathophysiological disease mechanisms.

Second, let us consider treatment of CRS and its impact on the inflammatory influx. The optimal treatment regime for CRS and NP at the moment comprises the use of nasal steroids either alone or in combination with a short treatment period with oral/systemic steroids. When samples of CRS or NP are collected at the time the patient is on the operating table it would seem clear that a significant bias will be introduced. Only those individuals that do not respond to treatment will be included in such a study, and it is unclear to what extent this population will be comparable with the general CRS or NP population. Taking the population under investigation off their medication will only partly remedy this caveat. Especially in treatment studies in which a group that will refrain from medication is compared with a group wherein technically, medication is reintroduced, one could argue that all differences detected between the treated and nontreated groups are potentially not relevant at all, as despite previous treatment these patients have remained symptomatic. It cannot be stressed enough that particularly this group of patients in whom medical treatment has failed would benefit most from a better understanding of the underlying disease, as a better understanding might lead to the discovery of new treatment options.

Third, consider other inflammatory diseases that are found as comorbidities in CRS. The most common of these must be allergy. This Th2 skewing disease is prevalent in Western society, and already for this reason alone one could expect a substantial part of the CRS population and the healthy controls to suffer from this additional inflammatory condition. In itself this will already murk the discussion whether in CRS one is dealing with a pure Th1, Th2, or mixed Th1/Th2 disease. Likewise, given that IL-5 and eosinophils are as important in allergy as they are thought to be in CRS and NP, the true extent of their involvement in CRS will be clouded. However, this issue can be even more severe as the distribution of allergy can vary enormously in the CRS population, or its effect cannot be judged at all, when no report is given on the prevalence of allergic disease in the studied populations. To prevent the possible caveat of comorbidities like allergy, it should be recommended only to compare CRS and NP in the absence of these comorbidities, or to compare patients with an allergic comorbidity with allergic individuals without CRS or NP.

Finally, the consequences of the selection of the samples used to study inflammation in CRS have to be considered. When one thinks of CRS as a general disease of the mucosa lining the (para)nasal sinuses, it may not matter whether a biopsy would be obtained from a turbinate or from a sinus. However, it is not clear whether all nasal mucosa or their inflammatory influx are identical, and one should caution that biopsies are taken only at easily accessible locations. In cases in which inflammation was studied at different locations, it was shown that polyp samples contain a significantly higher amount of eosinophils than the middle and inferior turbinate samples in the same NP patients, with a significantly higher number of eosinophils in the middle turbinate than in the inferior turbinate.[43–45] This result shows that in the case of NP one would need to be cautious in the characterization of an inflammatory influx, as a polyp structure is clearly different from CRS-affected diseased mucosa of a turbinate. Furthermore, in a comparison with healthy controls this could represent a significant bias, as polyps originate around the osteomeatal complex, material that is not easily collected from healthy individuals. However, the latter is not entirely impossible as patients with pituitary tumors are now often operated on endoscopically, and with the required removal of the sphenoid sinus, material from around the osteomeatal complex can be obtained in individuals who otherwise do not suffer from NP.

SUMMARY

Determining the inflammatory influx in CRS patients may yield a perhaps obvious benefit in addition to perhaps a more unexpected benefit. The first would be that how the inflammatory influx contributes to the pathogenesis of CRS and what toxic media-tors can be held responsible for the symptomatology would be better understood. A greater benefit could be that the makeup of the inflammatory influx in individual patients could be used more as a diagnostic tool that would complement the limited set of tools available to the clinician to determine the nature of the disease. Different subjective symptoms in patents, CT scans, and some objective measures to determine nasal patency in combination with a good anamnesis is all that can currently be used. Given that no symptom is truly unique for CRS or NP, and that different CRS patients may express different levels of symptoms, the task becomes even more difficult. However, on considering that the makeup of the cellular influx can be determined to a high level of detail, one might think of this makeup as defining the disease of that individual. This presumption might lead to grouping of patients based on their cellular influx, that in combination with the more traditional tools could lead to a better definition of CRS or to the identification of potential subgroups within CRS.

REFERENCES

1. Fokkens W, Lund V, Bachert C, et al. EAACI position paper on rhinosinusitis and nasal polyps executive summary. Allergy 2005;60:583–601 [Grade A].
2. European Academy of Allergology and Clinical Immunology taskforce. European position article on rhinosinusitis and nasal polyps. Rhinol Suppl 2005;18:1–87 [Grade A].
3. Fokkens W, Lund V, Mullol J, European Position Paper on Rhinosinusitis and Nasal Polyps group. European position paper on rhinosinusitis and nasal polyps 2007. European position paper on rhinosinusitis and nasal polyps. Rhinol Suppl 2007; 20:1–136 [Grade A].
4. Meltzer EO, Hamilos DL, Hadley JA, et al. Rhinosinusitis: establishing definitions for clinical research and patient care. J Allergy Clin Immunol 2004;114:155–212 [Grade A].
5. Bachert C, Van Bruaene N, Toskala E, et al. Important research questions in allergy and related diseases: 3-chronic rhinosinusitis and nasal polyposis— a GALEN study. Allergy 2009;64(4):520–33.
6. Ebbens FA, Maldonado M, de Groot EJ, et al. Topical glucocorticoids downre-gulate COX-1 positive cells in nasal polyps. Allergy 2009;64(1):96–103 [Grade A].
7. Mygind N, Dahl R, Bachert C. Nasal polyposis, eosinophil dominated inflamma-tion, and allergy. Thorax 2000;55(Suppl 2):S79–83.
8. Allen JS, Eisma R, La Freniere D. Characterization of the eosinophil chemokine RANTES in nasal polyps. Ann Otol Rhinol Laryngol 1998;107:416–20.

9. Bachert C, Hauser U, Prem B, et al. IL-5 synthesis is upregulated in human nasal polyp tissue. J Allergy Clin Immunol 1997;99:837–42.

10. Beck LA, Stellato C, Beall LD, et al. Detection of the chemokine RANTES and endothelial adhesion molecules in nasal polyps. J Allergy Clin Immunol 1996; 98:766–80.

11. Hamilos DL, Leung DY, Huston DP, et al. GM-CSF, IL-5 and RANTES immunore-activity and mRNA expression in chronic hyperplastic sinusitis with nasal polypo-sis (NP). Clin Exp Allergy 1998;28(9):1145–52.

12. Wei JL, Kita H, Sherris DA, et al. The chemotactic behavior of eosinophils in patients with chronic rhinosinusitis. Laryngoscope 2003;113(2):303–6.

13. Shin SH, Ponikau JU, Sherris DA, et al. Chronic rhinosinusitis: an enhanced immune response to ubiquitous airborne fungi. J Allergy Clin Immunol 2004;114(6):1369–75.

14. Ponikau JU, Sherris DA, Weaver A, et al. Treatment of chronic rhinosinusitis with intranasal amphotericin B: a randomized, placebo-controlled, double-blind pilot trial. J Allergy Clin Immunol 2005;115(1):125–31 [Grade B].

15. Ebbens FA, Georgalas C, Luiten S, et al. The effect of topical amphotericin B on inflammatory markers in patients with chronic rhinosinusitis: a multi-center randomized controlled study. Laryngoscope 2009;119(2):401–8.

16. Ebbens FA, Scadding GK, Badia L, et al. Amphotericin B nasal lavages: not a solution for patients with chronic rhinosinusitis. J Allergy Clin Immunol 2006; 118(5):1149–56 [Grade B].

17. Weschta M, Rimek D, Formanek M, et al. Topical antifungal treatment of chronic rhinosinusitis with nasal polyps: a randomized, double-blind clinical trial. J Allergy Clin Immunol 2004;113(6):1122–8 [Grade B].

18. Kountakis SE, Arango P, Bradley D, et al. Molecular and cellular staging for the severity of chronic rhinosinusitis. Laryngoscope 2004;114(11):1895–905.

19. Van Zele T, Claeys S, Gevaert P, et al. Differentiation of chronic sinus diseases by measurement of inflammatory mediators. Allergy 2006;61(11):1280–9.

20. Ebbens FA, Maldonado M, de Groot EJJ, et al. Cystic fibrosis nasal polyps: increased numbers of interleukin-5 expressing cells without marked tissue eosin-ophilia. In: Controversies in chronic rhinosinusitis. Thesis Ebbens FA. University of Amsterdam, the Netherlands; 2009. p. 57–69.

21. Zhang N, Van Zele T, Perez-Novo C, et al. Different types of T-effector cells orchestrate mucosal inflammation in chronic sinus disease. J Allergy Clin Immu-nol 2008;122(5):961–8.

22. Gevaert P, Lang-Loidolt D, Lackner A, et al. Nasal IL-5 levels determine the response to antiIL-5 treatment in patients with nasal polyps. J Allergy Clin Immu-nol 2006;118(5):1133–41 [Grade A].

23. Kostamo K, Sorsa T, Leino M, et al. In vivo relationship between collagenase-2 and interleukin-8 but not tumour necrosis factor-alpha in chronic rhinosinusitis with nasal polyposis. Allergy 2005;60(10):1275–9.

24. Chen YS, Arab SF, Westhofen M, et al. Expression of interleukin-5, interleukin-8, and interleukin-10 mRNA in the osteomeatal complex in nasal polyposis. Am J Rhinol 2005;19(2):117–23.

25. Ural A, Tezer MS, Yücel A, et al. Interleukin-4, interleukin-8 and E-selectin levels in intranasal polyposis patients with and without allergy: a comparative study. J Int Med Res 2006;34(5):520–4.

26. Ebbens FA, Rinia AB, Luiten S, et al. Increased neutrophil chemoattractant IL-8 is characteristic of all nasal polyp tissue specimens. In: Controversies in chronic rhi-nosinusitis. Thesis Ebbens FA. University of Amsterdam, the Netherlands; 2009. p. 29–40.

27. Romagnani S. Regulation of the T cell response. Clin Exp Allergy 2006;36:1357–66.
28. KleinJan A, Willart M, van Rijt LS, et al. An essential role for dendritic cells in human and experimental allergic rhinitis. J Allergy Clin Immunol 2006;118:1117–25.
29. Tang XL, Smith TR, Kumar V. Specific control of immunity by regulatory CD8 T cells. Cell Mol Immunol 2005;2:11–9.
30. Conley DB, Tripathi A, Seiberling KA, et al. Superantigens and chronic rhinosinusitis: skewing of T-cell receptor V beta-distributions in polyp-derived CD4+ and CD8+ T cells. Am J Rhinol 2006;20:534–9.
31. Conley DB, Tripathi A, Seiberling KA, et al. Superantigens and chronic rhinosinusitis II: analysis of T-cell receptor V beta domains in nasal polyps. Am J Rhinol 2006;20:451–5.
32. Gevaert P, Holtappels G, Johansson SG, et al. Organization of secondary lymphoid tissue and local IgE formation to *Staphylococcus aureus* enterotoxins in nasal polyp tissue. Allergy 2005;60:71–9.
33. Shoham T, Yaniv E, Koren R, et al. Reduced expression of activin A in focal lymphoid agglomerates within nasal polyps. J Histochem Cytochem 2001;49: 1245–52.
34. Rampey AM, Lathers DM, Woodworth BA, et al. Immunolocalization of dendritic cells and pattern recognition receptors in chronic rhinosinusitis. Am J Rhinol 2007;21:117–21.
35. Haas N, Hamann K, Grabbe J, et al. Demonstration of the high-affinity IgE receptor (Fc epsilon RI) on Langerhans' cells of diseased nasal mucosa. Allergy 1997;52:436–9.
36. Sanchez-Segura A, Brieva JA, Rodríguez C. T lymphocytes that infiltrate nasal polyps have a specialized phenotype and produce a mixed TH1/TH2 pattern of cytokines. J Allergy Clin Immunol 1998;102:953–60.
37. Laffón A, García-Vicuña R, Humbría A, et al. Upregulated expression and function of VLA-4 fibronectin receptors on human activated T cells in rheumatoid arthritis. J Clin Invest 1991;88:546–52.
38. Elhini A, Abdelwahab S, Ikeda K. Th1 and Th2 cell population in chronic ethmoidal rhinosinusitis: a chemokine receptor assay. Laryngoscope 2005;115:1272–7.
39. Syrbe U, Siveke J, Hamann A. Th1/Th2 subsets: distinct differences in homing and chemokine receptor expression? Springer Semin Immunopathol 1999;21:263–85.
40. Bernstein JM, Ballow M, Rich G, et al. Lymphocyte subpopulations and cytokines in nasal polyps: is there a local immune system in the nasal polyp? Otolanryngol Head and Neck Surgery 2004;130:526–35.
41. Van Bruaene N, Pérez-Novo CA, Basinski TM, et al. T-cell regulation in chronic paranasal sinus disease. J Allergy Clin Immunol 2008;121(6):1435–41.
42. Wang X, Dong Z, Zhu DD, et al. Expression profile of immune-associated genes in nasal polyps. Ann Otol Rhinol Laryngol 2006;115(6):450–6.
43. Stoop AE, van der Heijden HA, Biewenga J, et al. Eosinophils in nasal polyps and nasal mucosa: an immunohistochemical study. J Allergy Clin Immunol 1993;91: 616–22.
44. Jahnsen FL, Haraldsen G, Aanesen JP, et al. Eosinophil infiltration is related to increased expression of vascular cell adhesion molecule-1 in nasal polyps. Am J Respir Cell Mol Biol 1995;12:624–32.
45. Bernstein JM, Gorfien J, Noble B, et al. Nasal polyposis: immunohistochemistry and bioelectrical findings (a hypothesis for the development of nasal polyps). J Allergy Clin Immunol 1997;99:165–75.

Epithelium, Cilia, and Mucus: Their Importance in Chronic Rhinosinusitis

Marcelo B. Antunes, MD, David A. Gudis, MD, Noam A. Cohen, MD, PhD*

KEYWORDS

- Chronic rhinosinusitis • Mucociliary clearance • Cilia
- Mucus • Respiratory epithelium

Chronic rhinosinusitis (CRS), affecting more than 35 million Americans of all ages,[1] represents several distinct entities which are clinically indistinguishable. Although the mortality of the disease is low, the morbidity is high, with CRS patients demonstrating worse quality-of-life scores for physical pain and social functioning than those suffering from chronic obstructive pulmonary disease, congestive heart failure, or angina.[2] Multiple causes contribute to the development of CRS, but a common pathophysiologic sequela is ineffective sinonasal mucociliary clearance (MCC) due to impairment of 1 or more of its components (epithelium, cilia, and mucus) resulting in stasis of sinonasal secretions and subsequent chronic infection or persistent inflammation. Although the literature is contradictory regarding mucus viscosity,[3–5] and basal ciliary beat frequency (CBF)[4,6–9] in CRS, recent work has suggested that a subset of patients with CRS have a blunted ciliary response to environmental stimuli.[10] In addition, air-liquid interface cultures of respiratory epithelium from patients with CRS have demonstrated an increased transepithelial ion transport compared with normal cultures, thereby altering mucus viscosity and potentially contributing to the pathophysiology of the disease.[11]

This review discusses how the mucociliary components function and how their impairment may contribute to the development and progression of CRS.

EPITHELIUM

The sinonasal mucosa is lined by pseudostratified columnar ciliated epithelium. The epithelium has a variable number of ciliated cells ($\sim$75%), goblet cells ($\sim$20%), and basal cells ($\sim$5%), which reside on an acellular basement membrane (**Fig. 1**). This

Department of Otorhinolaryngology – Head and Neck Surgery, University of Pennsylvania School of Medicine, Ravdin Building 5th Floor, 3400 Spruce Street, Philadelphia, PA 19004, USA
* Corresponding author.
E-mail address: cohenn@uphs.upenn.edu (N.A. Cohen).

Immunol Allergy Clin N Am 29 (2009) 631–643
doi:10.1016/j.iac.2009.07.004
0889-8561/09/$ – see front matter © 2009 Elsevier Inc. All rights reserved.

immunology.theclinics.com

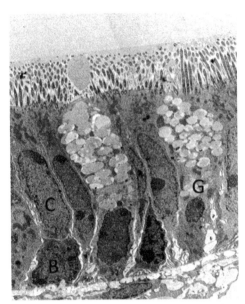

Fig. 1. Respiratory epithelium. Transmission electron microscopy demonstrating 3 cell types of the upper respiratory epithelium; G, goblet; C, ciliated; B, basal.

epithelial lining protects the upper airway from inhaled pathogens and debris by a process referred to as MCC and contributes to the innate immunity and antigen presentation defense mechanisms.[12]

The epithelium of each part of the nasal cavity is specialized to suit a particular region. In the anterior portion, the nasal vestibule, the epithelium is squamous stratified with sebaceous glands, sweat glands, vibrissa, and fine hair. The epithelium on this portion provides a barrier like the skin. At the nasal valves, a histologic transition occurs to the pseudostratified columnar ciliated epithelium. This epithelium is found throughout the sinonasal cavity with the exception of the olfactory epithelium.[13] Each ciliated epithelial cell of the sinonasal cavity has hundreds of motile cilia (discussed later) and even more immotile microvilli along its apical surface. The microvilli are thin hairlike projections of actin filaments, about 1 to 2 μm in length, covered by the cell membrane (**Fig. 2**, small arrow). The main function of microvilli is most likely to increase the apical surface area of the cell, thereby increasing the exchange process across the epithelium and optimizing secretory function. The microvilli also prevent drying of the surface by retaining moisture.[14] The ciliated epithelial cells contain numerous mitochondria (see **Fig. 2**, star) in the apical compartments generating the energy substrate necessary for the microvilli and cilia, as well as for secretory and transport function.

The goblet cells of the epithelium contribute to the respiratory secretions with the production of mucas. These cells contain secretory granules containing mucin, which is the principal component generating the elasticity and viscosity of the mucus layer. The apical surface of the goblet cell is also covered by microvilli and contains a small duct through which it releases the concentrated mucin (**Fig. 3**, black arrow). The mucus granules give the mature cell its shape, in which only a narrow portion of the basal cytoplasm touches the basement membrane (see **Fig. 1**G). There are no goblet cells in the squamous, transitional, or olfactory epithelium, and they are irregularly distributed throughout the sinonasal cavity. The basal cells are attached to the

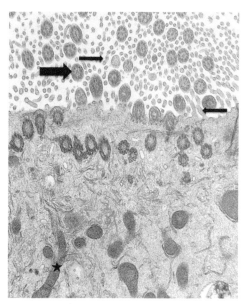

Fig. 2. Ciliated cell. Transmission electron microscopy of a sinonasal epithelial cell demonstrating cilia (*large arrow*) with the familiar 9 + 2 arrangement of microtubules as well as microvilli (*small black arrows*). In addition, the ciliated epithilial cell is packed with mitochondria for ATP synthesis (★)

basement membrane with no exposure to the apical surface of the epithelium, and thus are somewhat protected from the sinonasal cavity environment (see **Fig. 1**B). The basal cells have a dense cytoplasm with desmosomes, which promote adhesion between adjacent cells, and hemidesmosomes, which anchor the cell to the basement membrane. Basal cells are believed to serve as progenitor cells that can differentiate into goblet or ciliated cells,[15] although experiments with rat bronchial epithelium suggest that the primary progenitor cell is the nonciliated columnar population.[16] Basal cells are also believed to help in adhering the columnar cells to the basement membrane.

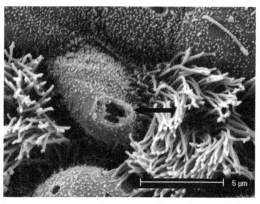

Fig. 3. Goblet cell. Scanning electron microscopy of a goblet cell demonstrating an open secretory duct as well as surface microvilli.

Sinonasal epithelial cells are connected through 3 types of intercellular junctions: adherens junctions bind cells to the basement membrane; tight junctions surround each epithelial cell and ensure impermeability of the epithelial layer to water, molecules, and pathogens; and gap junctions provide small windows communicating with the cytoplasm of adjacent cells, allowing ions and small signaling molecules to pass from one cell to the adjacent cell, thereby coordinating epithelial responses over epithelial microenvironments.[14] Below the basement membrane lies the lamina propria, a layer containing glands, vasculature, and nerves supplying the mucosa. The lamina propria is divided into a superficial glandular layer, a middle vascular layer, and a deep glandular layer. The glands of the lamina propria release mucus and serous secretions into the nasal cavity.

CILIA

Respiratory cilia clear the mucus blanket of pathogens and environmental debris from the upper and lower respiratory passages by beating in a coordinated and rhythmic manner. Cilia are cylindrical organelles protruding from the apical surface of epithelial cells, and are anchored by intracellular basal bodies derived from centrioles (**Fig. 4**). There are approximately 50 to 200 cilia per epithelial cell, each measuring 5 to 7 μm in length and 0.2 to 0.3 μm in diameter.[17,18] Each cilium consists of a bundle of interconnected microtubules, termed the axoneme, and an overlying membrane that is part of the cell plasma membrane. Microtubules are made of protofilaments, which in turn are composed of α- and β-tubulin dimers. The major β-tubulin in cilia is the type IV isotype,[19] which is much more abundant in the cilia than elsewhere in the cell and makes an ideal marker for respiratory cilia in the research setting.

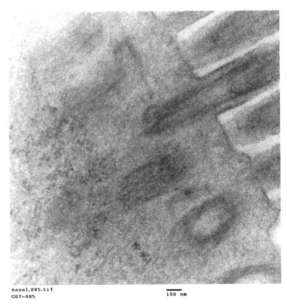

nasal.005.tif
G07-005   100 nm

Fig. 4. Basal body. Insertion of the cilia into the apical surface of the cell is anchored by the basal body, which determines the axis of the cilia, thereby defining the direction of the power and recovery strokes.

The axonemes of motile cilia contain 2 central singlet microtubules surrounded by 9 doublet microtubules. Each doublet consists of 1 α-tubule, a complete circle of 13 protofilaments, and 1 β-tubule, an incomplete circle of 10 protofilaments. This axoneme structure is preserved across the motile cilia of the respiratory epithelium, oviduct, and ventricular ependymal cells. The 2 central microtubules are attached by paired bridges, whereas the peripheral doublets attach to the central pair via radial spoke heads. Each outer doublet interacts with the adjacent outer doublets via inner dynein arms (IDAs), outer dynein arms (ODAs), and nexin, each having a distinct role in the dynamic motion of cilia bending.[20] Activation of the dynein arms generates a sliding motion of 1 microtubule doublet against the adjacent doublet. Phosphorylation of the ODAs regulates cilia beat frequency, whereas phosphorylation of the IDAs regulates the wave form pattern of beating.[21,22] Although the function of the radial spoke heads is not entirely understood, it seems they are involved in regionally limiting the sliding between the microtubules during the ciliary stroke, thus converting the sliding motion generated by the dynein arms into a bending motion of the axoneme.[23]

Each cilium has a forward power stroke followed by a recovery stroke. During the power stroke the cilium is fully extended, and, at the apogee of the arc, the distal tip makes contact with the viscous outer mucus layer (gel phase), thereby transmitting directional force to the overlying mucus blanket. During the recovery stroke, the cilium bends 90° and sweeps back to its starting point within the thinner periciliary fluid layer (sol phase). The mechanism of ciliary motion depends on a series of ATP-dependent molecular motors that cause the outer doublets of the axoneme to slide relative to each other, producing a vectorial force. The central pair of microtubule singlets divides the axoneme into 2 opposing halves. As proposed by the "switch point" hypothesis, the dynein motors on 1 side of the axoneme are predominantly active during the effective stroke, whereas the motors on the other side are mainly active during the recovery stroke.[24] If the microtubules are numbered in a clockwise fashion from 1 to 9, the effective stroke would involve the ODAs on the 9-1-2-3-4 microtubules, and the recovery stroke would involve activity of the dynein in the 5-6-7-8 microtubules.[25] The dynamic force of each power stroke is directly proportional to the number of dynein-microtubule interactions,[26] and there is usually a physiologic reserve available to increase the force of the stroke when necessary.[27] The orientation of the stroke is determined by the orientation of the anchoring basal body of the axoneme.[28,29]

Although it is well established that cilia beat in a coordinated fashion, referred to as a metachronous wave, the mechanism of coordination is not entirely understood. One theory to explain the coordinated wavelike motion of cilia is that gap junctions connecting adjacent epithelial cells may allow a directional propagation of intracellular calcium or waves driving the microtubule interactions and ultimately the entire metachronous wave.[30] Inositol triphosphate (IP3) has also been demonstrated to coordinate ciliary beating.[31] Another possible mechanism relies on the close relationship between the cilia and the hydrodynamic forces surrounding them in their partly liquid environment, in which only a small number of coordinated cilia would be necessary to generate a hydrodynamic wave that, in turn, would force the timed coordinating beating of nearby cilia.[32] Once a metachronous wave is established, spontaneous beating can range from approximately 9 to 15 Hz in humans, with ciliary tip velocities of 600 to 1000 μm/s. The resultant dynamic range of mucus velocity is about 50 μm/s to 450 μm/s, or 3 mm/min to 25 mm/min. The power and speed of the cilia result in a highly efficient mechanism that can clear the mucus blanket of the entire nose or sinus in 10 minutes.[33]

CBF changes in response to several other chemical,[34,35] thermal,[36,37] mechanical,[38–40] and hormonal[41–43] stimuli. Small changes in extracellular and intracellular pH can have a profound impact on CBF. An increase in intracellular pH produces an increase in CBF, whereas a decrease in pH produces a decrease in CBF.[44] However, it is not known whether this effect is due to modulation of kinase activity, even though an acidic pH has been demonstrated to inhibit PKA function,[45] or by directly regulating the ODAs of the axoneme.[46] CBF has also been shown to vary directly with temperature, with the ideal temperature for CBF being from 32 to 37°C.[36,37,47] Furthermore, direct mechanical stimulation of the cilia promotes an increase in CBF which coincides with an increase in intracellular Ca^{2+}.[40]

Extracellular nucleotides (adenosine and uridine) are especially potent regulators of epithelial functions that stimulate MCC in several ways. These nucleotides are released by local epithelium in response to mechanical and osmotic stimuli and act in a paracrine fashion.[38] Through metabotropic and ionotropic receptors, the nucleotides increase mucus secretion, increase CBF, and gate ion channels involved in maintaining epithelial surface liquid volume.[48] This capability generates a tremendous reserve for dynamic regulation of MCC when the respiratory system is environmentally challenged or stimulated.

Furthermore, adrenergic,[43,49,50] cholinergic,[51,52] and peptidergic[53,54] stimulation have also been demonstrated to stimulate ciliary motility. These environmental and host stimuli are transmitted via surface receptors and channels to trigger activation of second messenger cascades that regulate phosphorylation status of ciliary proteins, thereby modulating the kinetics of microtubules sliding relative to each other. IP_3-mediated calcium transients have been correlated with increased CBF.[31,55–57] Additionally, protein kinase A (PKA),[52,58] protein kinase G (PKG),[59,60] and a nitric oxide (NO)-dependent mechanisms of CBF stimulation have been proposed,[35,61,62] whereas activation of protein kinase C (PKC) seems to decrease CBF.[54,63] To maintain rapid control of ciliary activity, kinase anchoring proteins (AKAPs), kinases, and phosphatases have been demonstrated to be tightly associated with the axoneme.[64–66]

MUCUS

The sinonasal epithelium is covered by a mucus blanket with dynamic properties. When aerosolized pathogens and particles larger than 0.5 to 1 μm pass through the nasal cavities they become entrapped in this mucus layer. Through the beating action of the cilia, the debris laden mucus is propelled to the pharynx where it is swallowed.

The mucus consists of 2 layers: a continuous inner sol phase of lower viscosity, comprised of water and electrolytes, which surrounds the cilia shafts; and a discontinuous outer gel phase of higher viscosity, which rides along the tips of the extended cilia. The mucus layer is immunologically active, being composed of water (95%), peptides, salts, and debris, having a slightly acidic pH of 5.5 to 6.5.[17] Approximately 600 to 1800 mL of mucus are generated every day.[67]

The sources of nasal secretions are multiple and include anterior nasal glands, submucosal glands, epithelial glands (goblet cells), lacrimal secretions, and transudate from the rich capillary vasculature. Mucin proteins consist of a group of large glycoproteins with peptide backbones and oligosaccharide side chains. The mucins generate the rheologic properties of viscosity and elasticity that characterize the respiratory mucus. As mentioned earlier, mucins are secreted by goblet cells in a condensed form and undergo hydration to form a gel, creating this unique fluid structure that facilitates MCC, enhancing the clearing of entrapped debris. In addition to generating a medium for trapping foreign inhaled material, the mucins contribute to the respiratory host defense in other ways. Mucins can bind to surface adhesins on microorganisms. The recognition of these surface adhesions have been identified on *Mycoplasma pneumoniae*, *Streptococcus pneumoniae*, *Pseudomonas aeruginosa*, influenza virus and *Escherichia coli*.[68] This specific adhesivity provides additional protection in the sense that there is strengthening of the bond between the microorganisms and the mucus optimizing the clearance. Mucins may also bind other innate immune proteins such as lactoferrin and lysozyme, facilitating their role in the immune response.[69] In addition, immunoglobulins, surfactants, and antitrypsin contribute to the immunologic role of mucus. Transudation increases in pathologic processes, increasing the periciliary layer depth and impairing MCC. This process has been described in allergic rhinitis, in which nasal washes demonstrate elevated levels of albumin after provocation.[70] The mucus rafts move as a result of the motion of the periciliary fluid and the contact of the ciliary tips with the plaques. Therefore, if there is an increase in the periciliary layer, the ciliary tips will fail to reach the mucus rafts, and the periciliary layer movement will be the only means to propel the mucus.

SINONASAL MCC PATTERNS

As remarkable as the ability of microscopic cilia to create coordinated waves and propel mucus is their ability to orient their motion, to direct the mucus toward its macroscopic anatomic destination. The mucus of the paranasal sinuses is directed toward the nasal cavity, where it then traverses to the posterior nasopharynx and is eventually ingested. Appreciation of the natural clearance patterns of the sinuses is critical for successful surgical intervention, especially the frontal sinus, as scarring of confluence regions may lead to mucostasis.

In the maxillary sinus, mucus must flow superiorly, against gravity, from the most inferior portion of the cavity. It courses upward along the walls of the entire cavity and then toward the natural ostium in the superior medial wall of the sinus, which drains into the ethmoidal infundibulum. The mucus that courses along the lateral wall of the maxillary sinus is carried medially along the sinus roof to reach the ostium. The anterior ethmoid cells direct their mucus toward their individual ostia, then into the middle meatus, whereas the posterior ethmoid cells direct their mucus toward the superior meatus and eventually into the sphenoethmoidal recess. The sphenoid sinus also directs its mucus toward its natural ostium and then into the sphenoethmoidal recess. The mucus flow pattern in the frontal sinus seems to be unique in that it demonstrates retrograde and antegrade motion. Mucus along the medial portion of the sinus is carried superiorly, away from the ostium, and then laterally along the roof of the sinus. The mucus along the floor and the inferior portions of the anterior and posterior walls is then carried medially toward the ostium, where it drains from the frontal recess into the infundibulum.[71]

The mucociliary flow from the anterior sinuses converges at the osteomeatal complex, where the mucus is carried via the uncinate process and inferior turbinate to the posterior nasopharynx, generally passing anteriorly and inferiorly to the eustachian tube orifice. The mucociliary flow from the posterior sinuses, however, tends to travel to the posterior nasopharynx posteriorly and superiorly to the eustachian tube orifice.[71] Once in the posterior nasopharynx, further ciliary motion and swallowing direct the mucus blanket into the gastrointestinal tract, where infectious pathogens are far less likely to survive and cause infection.

CRS

MCC is dependent on normal cilia function and mucus composition. Thus disease states that compromise this essential mode of defense tend to result in impaired clearance of infectious pathogens and ultimately recurrent sinopulmonary infections. When one or more of those components (epithelium, cilia, and mucus) do not function appropriately, the respiratory secretions stagnate and ultimately harbor infection resulting in inflammation. In time this becomes a chronic inflammatory state that persists with or without active infection. Several disease processes have been recognized in which 1 of those components does not work, resulting in chronic sinusitis.

Cystic fibrosis (CF) is an autosomal recessive disorder involving several organ systems that is caused by a single gene mutation resulting in defective electrolyte transport and, subsequently, abnormal mucus secretion.[72] The defect is in the cystic fibrosis transmembrane regulator (CFTR), a cAMP-mediated membrane glycoprotein that forms a chloride channel and intimately regulates the opening probability of sodium channels (ENaC).[73] The movement of intracellular water from the endothelium into the extracellular mucus layer is an osmotic process that follows electrolyte concentrations. Therefore, patients with defective sodium chloride transport develop abnormally viscous mucus. The goblet cells become engorged and distended. These patients have severely impaired MCC and frequently develop severe recurrent sinopulmonary infections.[74]

Upper respiratory infections, inflammation, mucosal swelling, and anatomic anomalies may disrupt the normal mucus composition or MCC flow pattern. When obstruction occurs in key areas like the osteomeatal complex or eustachian tube orifice, associated symptomatology commonly results. Ciliary motion can, however, adapt to a dynamic landscape, such as by transporting the mucus blanket around changing irregularities such as septal spurs.[75]

Primary ciliary dyskinesia (PCD), or immotile cilia syndrome, is an inherited disorder of dysfunctional cilia that manifests as severely impaired MCC. PCD patients typically present with chronic airway and recurrent middle ear infections. Because embryonic nodal cilia, essential for the normal left-right asymmetry of visceral development, are likewise defective, approximately 50% of PCD patients have situs inversus.[76] Many patients, men and women, also suffer from infertility because sperm motility and fallopian tube transport of ova depend on functional cilia. Kartagener syndrome is a subgroup of PCD marked by the triad of chronic sinusitis, situs inversus, and bronchiectasis. The diagnosis is usually suspected in children with recurrent episodes of otitis, sinusitis, pneumonia, and bronchiectais, and is confirmed by electron microscopy examination of the cilia structure. The original description of the inherited defect is in the dynein arms of axonemal microtubules which may result in the absence of the ODA, the IDA, or both. Other defects have been characterized and include complete or partial absence of radial spokes, and an abnormal number or configuration of microtubules. Other subsets of PCD patients may demonstrate normal ciliary structure but random ciliary orientation. Thus, despite normal motility, cilia function is ineffective and results in impaired MCC.[77]

In addition to inherited pathologies, exposure to various environmental pathogens can alter the normal MCC system. Infectious organisms that can interfere with their host's mucociliary defense have a survival advantage, and several have indeed adapted such mechanisms. Common bacterial pathogens such as *Haemophilus influenzae*, *Streptococcus pneumoniae*, *Staphylococcus aureus*, and *Pseudomonas* produce specific toxins to impair ciliary motion and coordination.[78] Viruses responsible for common upper respiratory infections disrupt the microtubule function of ciliated columnar cells and change the viscosity of surrounding mucus.[75] Impairing the local defense system facilitates colonization of the upper airway by infectious pathogens.

ASSESSMENT OF MCC IN PATIENTS WITH CRS

Most assessments of MCC are performed using 1 of 2 techniques: measurement of MCC time by applying a substance in the tissue and following its clearance, or by measurement of CBF.

Mucociliary Transport in CRS

Several investigators studied MCC in patients with chronic sinusitis. Most studies demonstrated that clearance in patients with chronic sinusitis is slower than in healthy controls.[6,79,80] In a related study 1 investigator attempted to elucidate the contribution of ciliary function abnormality versus mucus abnormalities in the slow clearance that was observed.[4] The investigators removed mucus from patients with chronic sinusitis and healthy subjects and placed it into a frog's palate. Mucociliary transport in the frog's palate was not different among the different groups, suggesting that factors other than the rheologic properties of the mucus control MCC velocity. More recently, elegant culturing techniques, termed air-liquid interface cultures, have been established from patients with CRS and using short-circuit recordings have demonstrated an increased transepithelial ion transport compared with normal cultures, thereby altering mucus viscosity and potentially contributing to the pathophysiology of the disease.[11]

CBF

As discussed earlier in cilia function, respiratory cilia have an intrinsic basal frequency and the ability to increase beat frequency following stimulation. Investigations assessing CBF in CRS have predominately focused on the basal frequency and have reported conflicting results, with some studies indicating depressed basal frequency, whereas others demonstrated no alterations between CRS patients and non-CRS patients.[4,6–10] Recently, work focusing on the ability of the cilia to respond to stimulation has suggested that a subset of patients with CRS have a blunted ciliary response to environmental stimuli.[10] This blunted response was not permanent,[81] but was reversible, reflecting the ability of patients appropriately treated for CRS to normalize their mucociliary transport time.

SUMMARY

The entire respiratory system is constantly exposed to environmental pollutants, respiratory pathogens, and aerosolized toxins. MCC is the primary innate defense mechanism against this constant onslaught. During the last quarter of a century techniques to study MCC, and the individual components, cilia and mucus, have evolved. These techniques have advanced our understanding of the interaction of the respiratory epithelium with the airway surface liquid, and have begun to shed light on the pathologic ramifications of subtle alterations in the homeostasis of MCC. Additional work on alterations of sinonasal respiratory epithelial cell function will undoubtedly lead to a more comprehensive understanding of the disease processes involved in the CRS syndrome and result in improved therapeutic interventions.

REFERENCES

1. Murphy MP, Fishman P, Short SO, et al. Health care utilization and cost among adults with chronic rhinosinusitis enrolled in a health maintenance organization. Otolaryngol Head Neck Surg 2002;127(5):367–76.

2. Gliklich RE, Metson R. The health impact of chronic sinusitis in patients seeking otolaryngologic care. Otolaryngol Head Neck Surg 1995;113(1):104–9.

3. Majima Y, Harada T, Shimizu T, et al. Effect of biochemical components on rheologic properties of nasal mucus in chronic sinusitis. Am J Respir Crit Care Med 1999;160(2):421–6.

4. Majima Y, Sakakura Y, Matsubara T, et al. Possible mechanisms of reduction of nasal mucociliary clearance in chronic sinusitis. Clin Otolaryngol 1986;11(2):55–60.

5. Atsuta S, Majima Y. Nasal mucociliary clearance of chronic sinusitis in relation to rheological properties of nasal mucus. Ann Otol Rhinol Laryngol 1998;107(1):47–51.

6. Majima Y, Sakakura Y, Matsubara T, et al. Mucociliary clearance in chronic sinusitis: related human nasal clearance and in vitro bullfrog palate clearance. Biorheology 1983;20(2):251–62.

7. Joki S, Toskala E, Saano V, et al. Correlation between ciliary beat frequency and the structure of ciliated epithelia in pathologic human nasal mucosa. Laryngoscope 1998;108(3):426–30.

8. Braverman I, Wright ED, Wang CG, et al. Human nasal ciliary-beat frequency in normal and chronic sinusitis subjects. J Otolaryngol 1998;27(3):145–52.

9. Nuutinen J, Rauch-Toskala E, Saano V, et al. Ciliary beating frequency in chronic sinusitis. Arch Otolaryngol Head Neck Surg 1993;119(6):645–7.

10. Chen B, Shaari J, Claire SE, et al. Altered sinonasal ciliary dynamics in chronic rhinosinusitis. Am J Rhinol 2006;20(3):325–9.

11. Dejima K, Randell SH, Stutts MJ, et al. Potential role of abnormal ion transport in the pathogenesis of chronic sinusitis. Arch Otolaryngol Head Neck Surg 2006;132(12):1352–62.

12. Schleimer RP, Kato A, Kern R, et al. Epithelium: at the interface of innate and adaptive immune responses. J Allergy Clin Immunol 2007;120(6):1279–84.

13. Wagenmann M, Naclerio RM. Anatomic and physiologic considerations in sinusitis. J Allergy Clin Immunol 1992;90(3 Pt 2):419–23.

14. Busse WW, Holgate ST. Asthma and rhinitis. 2nd edition. Oxford; Malden (MA): Blackwell Science; 2000.

15. Eliezer N, Sade J, Silberberg A, et al. The role of mucus in transport by cilia. Am Rev Respir Dis 1970;102(1):48–52.

16. Evans MJ, Shami SG, Cabral-Anderson LJ, et al. Role of nonciliated cells in renewal of the bronchial epithelium of rats exposed to NO_2. Am J Pathol 1986;123(1):126–33.

17. Houtmeyers E, Gosselink R, Gayan-Ramirez G, et al. Regulation of mucociliary clearance in health and disease. Eur Respir J 1999;13(5):1177–88.

18. Satir P, Sleigh MA. The physiology of cilia and mucociliary interactions. Annu Rev Physiol 1990;52:137–55.

19. Renthal R, Schneider BG, Miller MM, et al. Beta IV is the major beta-tubulin isotype in bovine cilia. Cell Motil Cytoskeleton 1993;25(1):19–29.

20. Hard R, Blaustein K, Scarcello L. Reactivation of outer-arm-depleted lung axonemes: evidence for functional differences between inner and outer dynein arms in situ. Cell Motil Cytoskeleton 1992;21(3):199–209.

21. Brokaw CJ. Control of flagellar bending: a new agenda based on dynein diversity. Cell Motil Cytoskeleton 1994;28(3):199–204.

22. Brokaw CJ, Kamiya R. Bending patterns of *Chlamydomonas* flagella: IV. Mutants with defects in inner and outer dynein arms indicate differences in dynein arm function. Cell Motil Cytoskeleton 1987;8(1):68–75.

23. Satir P, Christensen ST. Overview of structure and function of mammalian cilia. Annu Rev Physiolog 2007;69:377–400.
24. Satir P, Matsuoka T. Splitting the ciliary axoneme: implications for a "switch-point" model of dynein arm activity in ciliary motion. Cell Motil Cytoskeleton 1989;14(3): 345–58.
25. Sanderson MJ, Sleigh MA. Ciliary activity of cultured rabbit tracheal epithelium: beat pattern and metachrony. J Cell Sci 1981;47:331–47.
26. Holwill ME, Foster GF, Hamasaki T, et al. Biophysical aspects and modelling of ciliary motility. Cell Motil Cytoskeleton 1995;32(2):114–20.
27. Johnson NT, Villalon M, Royce FH, et al. Autoregulation of beat frequency in respiratory ciliated cells. Demonstration by viscous loading. Am Rev Respir Dis 1991; 144(5):1091–4.
28. Satir P. The cilium as a biological nanomachine. FASEB J 1999;13(Suppl 2): S235–7.
29. Lee CH, Lee SS, Mo JH, et al. Comparison of ciliary wave disorders measured by image analysis and electron microscopy. Acta Otolaryngol 2005;125(5):571–6.
30. Yeh TH, Su MC, Hsu CJ, et al. Epithelial cells of nasal mucosa express functional gap junctions of connexin 43. Acta Otolaryngol 2003;123(2):314–20.
31. Barrera NP, Morales B, Villalon M. Plasma and intracellular membrane inositol 1,4,5-trisphosphate receptors mediate the $Ca(2+)$ increase associated with the ATP-induced increase in ciliary beat frequency. Am J Physiol Cell Physiol 2004; 287(4):C1114–24.
32. Gheber L, Priel Z. Synchronization between beating cilia. Biophys J 1989;55(1): 183–91.
33. Hilding AC. The role of the respiratory mucosa in health and disease. Minn Med 1967;50(6):915–9.
34. Wong LB, Miller IF, Yeates DB. Stimulation of tracheal ciliary beat frequency by capsaicin. J Appl Physiol 1990;68(6):2574–80.
35. Jain B, Rubinstein I, Robbins RA, et al. Modulation of airway epithelial cell ciliary beat frequency by nitric oxide. Biochem Biophys Res Commun 1993;191(1):83–8.
36. Mwimbi XK, Muimo R, Green MW, et al. Making human nasal cilia beat in the cold: a real time assay for cell signalling. Cell Signal 2003;15(4):395–402.
37. Schipor I, Palmer JN, Cohen AS, et al. Quantification of ciliary beat frequency in sinonasal epithelial cells using differential interference contrast microscopy and high-speed digital video imaging. Am J Rhinol 2006;20(1):124–7.
38. Winters SL, Davis CW, Boucher RC. Mechanosensitivity of mouse tracheal ciliary beat frequency: roles for Ca^{2+}, purinergic signaling, tonicity, and viscosity. Am J Physiol Lung Cell Mol Physiol 2007;292:L614–24.
39. Andrade YN, Fernandes J, Vazquez E, et al. TRPV4 channel is involved in the coupling of fluid viscosity changes to epithelial ciliary activity. J Cell Biol 2005; 168(6):869–74.
40. Sanderson MJ, Dirksen ER. Mechanosensitivity of cultured ciliated cells from the mammalian respiratory tract: implications for the regulation of mucociliary transport. Proc Natl Acad Sci U S A 1986;83(19):7302–6.
41. Jain B, Rubinstein I, Robbins RA, et al. TNF-alpha and IL-1 beta upregulate nitric oxide-dependent ciliary motility in bovine airway epithelium. Am J Physiol 1995; 268(6 Pt 1):L911–7.
42. Korngreen A, Ma W, Priel Z, et al. Extracellular ATP directly gates a cation-selective channel in rabbit airway ciliated epithelial cells. J Physiol 1998;508(Pt 3): 703–20.

43. Sanderson MJ, Dirksen ER. Mechanosensitive and beta-adrenergic control of the ciliary beat frequency of mammalian respiratory tract cells in culture. Am Rev Respir Dis 1989;139(2):432–40.

44. Sutto Z, Conner GE, Salathe M. Regulation of human airway ciliary beat frequency by intracellular pH. J Physiol 2004;560(Pt 2):519–32.

45. Reddy MM, Kopito RR, Quinton PM. Cytosolic pH regulates GCl through control of phosphorylation states of CFTR. Am J Physiol 1998;275(4 Pt 1):C1040–7.

46. Keskes L, Giroux-Widemann V, Serres C, et al. The reactivation of demembranated human spermatozoa lacking outer dynein arms is independent of pH. Mol Reprod Dev 1998;49(4):416–25.

47. Green A, Smallman LA, Logan AC, et al. The effect of temperature on nasal ciliary beat frequency. Clin Otolaryngol 1995;20(2):178–80.

48. Picher M, Boucher RC. Human airway ecto-adenylate kinase. A mechanism to propagate ATP signaling on airway surfaces. J Biol Chem 2003;278(13):11256–64.

49. Wyatt TA, Sisson JH. Chronic ethanol downregulates PKA activation and ciliary beating in bovine bronchial epithelial cells. Am J Physiol Lung Cell Mol Physiol 2001;281(3):L575–81.

50. Yang B, Schlosser RJ, McCaffrey TV. Dual signal transduction mechanisms modulate ciliary beat frequency in upper airway epithelium. Am J Physiol 1996;270(5 Pt 1):L745–51.

51. Salathe M, Lipson EJ, Ivonnet PI, et al. Muscarinic signaling in ciliated tracheal epithelial cells: dual effects on Ca2+ and ciliary beating. Am J Physiol 1997;272(2 Pt 1):L301–10.

52. Zagoory O, Braiman A, Priel Z. The mechanism of ciliary stimulation by acetylcholine: roles of calcium, PKA, and PKG. J Gen Physiol 2002;119(4):329–39.

53. Wong LB, Miller IF, Yeates DB. Pathways of substance P stimulation of canine tracheal ciliary beat frequency. J Appl Physiol 1991;70(1):267–73.

54. Wong LB, Park CL, Yeates DB. Neuropeptide Y inhibits ciliary beat frequency in human ciliated cells via nPKC, independently of PKA. Am J Physiol 1998;275(2 Pt 1):C440–8.

55. Salathe M, Bookman RJ. Coupling of [Ca2+]i and ciliary beating in cultured tracheal epithelial cells. J Cell Sci 1995;108(Pt 2):431–40.

56. Korngreen A, Priel Z. Simultaneous measurement of ciliary beating and intracellular calcium. Biophys J 1994;67(1):377–80.

57. Lansley AB, Sanderson MJ. Regulation of airway ciliary activity by Ca2+: simultaneous measurement of beat frequency and intracellular Ca2+. Biophys J 1999;77(1):629–38.

58. Braiman A, Zagoory O, Priel Z. PKA induces Ca2+ release and enhances ciliary beat frequency in a Ca2+-dependent and -independent manner. Am J Physiol 1998;275(3 Pt 1):C790–7.

59. Zhang L, Sanderson MJ. The role of cGMP in the regulation of rabbit airway ciliary beat frequency. J Physiol 2003;551(Pt 3):765–76.

60. Wyatt TA, Spurzem JR, May K, et al. Regulation of ciliary beat frequency by both PKA and PKG in bovine airway epithelial cells. Am J Physiol 1998;275(4 Pt 1):L827–35.

61. Yang B, Schlosser RJ, McCaffrey TV. Signal transduction pathways in modulation of ciliary beat frequency by methacholine. Ann Otol Rhinol Laryngol 1997;106(3):230–6.

62. Uzlaner N, Priel Z. Interplay between the NO pathway and elevated [Ca2+]i enhances ciliary activity in rabbit trachea. J Physiol 1999;516(Pt 1):179–90.

63. Mwimbi XK, Muimo R, Green M, et al. Protein kinase C regulates the flow rate-dependent decline in human nasal ciliary beat frequency in vitro. J Aerosol Med 2000;13(3):273–9.

64. Porter ME, Sale WS. The 9 + 2 axoneme anchors multiple inner arm dyneins and a network of kinases and phosphatases that control motility. J Cell Biol 2000; 151(5):F37–42.

65. Kamiya R. Functional diversity of axonemal dyneins as studied in *Chlamydomonas* mutants. Int Rev Cytol 2002;219:115–55.

66. Smith EF. Regulation of flagellar dynein by the axonemal central apparatus. Cell Motil Cytoskeleton 2002;52(1):33–42.

67. Tos M. Mucous elements in the nose. Rhinology 1976;14(4):155–62.

68. Adkinson NF, Middleton E. Middleton's allergy: principles & practice. 6th edition. St. Louis: Mosby; 2003.

69. Lamblin G, Aubert JP, Perini JM, et al. Human respiratory mucins. Eur Respir J 1992;5(2):247–56.

70. Baumgarten CR, Togias AG, Naclerio RM, et al. Influx of kininogens into nasal secretions after antigen challenge of allergic individuals. J Clin Invest 1985; 76(1):191–7.

71. Donald PJ, Gluckman JL, Rice DH. The sinuses. New York: Raven Press; 1995.

72. Accurso FJ. Update in cystic fibrosis 2005. Am J Respir Crit Care Med 2006; 173(9):944–7.

73. Wine JJ. The genesis of cystic fibrosis lung disease. J Clin Invest 1999;103(3): 309–12.

74. Van de Water TR, Staecker H. Otolaryngology: basic science and clinical review. New York: Thieme; 2005.

75. Jones N. The nose and paranasal sinuses physiology and anatomy. Adv Drug Deliv Rev 2001;51(1–3):5–19.

76. Noone PG, Leigh MW, Sannuti A, et al. Primary ciliary dyskinesia: diagnostic and phenotypic features. Am J Respir Crit Care Med 2004;169(4):459–67.

77. Rutland J, de Iongh RU. Random ciliary orientation. A cause of respiratory tract disease. N Engl J Med 1990;323(24):1681–4.

78. Ferguson JL, McCaffrey TV, Kern EB, et al. The effects of sinus bacteria on human ciliated nasal epithelium in vitro. Otolaryngol Head Neck Surg 1988;98(4): 299–304.

79. Wilson R, Sykes DA, Currie D, et al. Beat frequency of cilia from sites of purulent infection. Thorax 1986;41(6):453–8.

80. Passali D, Ferri R, Becchini G, et al. Alterations of nasal mucociliary transport in patients with hypertrophy of the inferior turbinates, deviations of the nasal septum and chronic sinusitis. Eur Arch Otorhinolaryngol 1999;256(7):335–7.

81. Chen B, Antunes MB, Claire SE, et al. Reversal of chronic rhinosinusitis-associated sinonasal ciliary dysfunction. Am J Rhinol 2007;21(3):346–53.

Are Biofilms the Answer in the Pathophysiology and Treatment of Chronic Rhinosinusitis?

Shaun J. Kilty, MD[a], Martin Y. Desrosiers, MD[b,c],*

KEYWORDS

- Biofilms • Chronic sinusitis • Endoscopic sinus surgery
- Staphylococcus aureus • Pseudomonas aeruginosa
- Coagulase-negative staphylococci • Haemophilus influenzae
- Biofilm therapy

Although the discovery of a bacterial biofilm is centuries old, it was not until recently that evidence for bacterial biofilm formation and control was found.[1–3] Since then, there has been an intensive development of scientific knowledge of biofilm growth, behavior, and therapy. In otolaryngology, a great deal of knowledge has developed implicating bacterial biofilms in recurrent adenotonsillar infection, otitis media, cholesteatoma, and chronic rhinosinusitis (CRS).[4,5] To date, rhinologic research on biofilm disease in CRS suggests that biofilms may significantly contribute to the chronic inflammation that is characteristic of this disease. How central a role they play remains the subject of debate.

WHAT IS A BIOFILM?

A biofilm is an organized community of bacteria adherent to a mucosal surface or foreign body, situated in an extensive extracellular polymeric substance (EPS, or glycocalyx) composed primarily of polysaccharides, but also containing protein and

[a] Department of Otolaryngology- Head and Neck Surgery, University of Ottawa, Ottawa Hospital, Civic Campus, 1053 Carling Avenue, Ottawa, Ontario K1Y 4E9, Canada
[b] Department of Otolaryngology, Hôpital Hôtel-Dieu, Pavillon Hôtel-Dieu, Université de Montréal, 3840, rue St Urbain, Montreal, Quebec H2W 1T8, Canada
[c] Department of Otolaryngology, McGill University, 687 Pine Avenue West Montreal, Quebec H3A 1A1, Canada
* Corresponding author. Department of Otolaryngology, Pavillon Hôtel-Dieu, 3840, rue St Urbain, Montreal, QC H2W 1T8, Canada.
E-mail address: desrosiers_martin@hotmail.com (M.Y. Desrosiers).

Immunol Allergy Clin N Am 29 (2009) 645–656
doi:10.1016/j.iac.2009.07.005
0889-8561/09/$ – see front matter © 2009 Elsevier Inc. All rights reserved.

DNA.[6] The glycocalyx is a mixture of bacterial colonies of various phenotypes with different physiochemical properties. It serves as protection for its bacterial inhabitants while also modulating the microenvironment of the colonies through its numerous water channels via a process of interbacterial signaling called quorum sensing.[6]

Bacterial biofilms appear to be relevant in chronic or in complex infections. When in the form of a biofilm, infectious bacteria are difficult to detect and culture using conventional methods and are largely resistant to current antimicrobial therapy. This marked resistance to antibiotic therapy was previously believed to be secondary to a mechanically protective effect of the coating; however, new studies document that antibiotics freely penetrate the bacterial biofilm and that resistance is probably more related to slow growth conditions within the biofilm and sharing of multiple resistance genes within the members of the biofilm community.

To date, the identification of a biofilm has relied on the analysis of tissue samples directly with electron or confocal scanning laser microscopy (CSLM) or indirectly by identification of a DNA signature for presence of biofilm-forming genes (**Figs. 1–4**). No simple, noninvasive clinical test for detecting biofilms is currently available. In a similar vein, there are no medical treatments that specifically target biofilms in the human host.

Biofilm Development

The formation of a bacterial biofilm is composed of several concurrent steps. For biofilm to form, a nutrient-rich microenvironment must be present to allow for the survival and replication of the biofilm-initiating planktonic organisms. This microenvironment is provided by essentially all bodily fluids. Some environments, such as endothelial or epithelial surfaces, may be more resistant to biofilm initiation because of their innate antimicrobial defenses and, in some cases, by the symbiotic native bacteria biofilms that inhibit the adhesion of other planktonic organisms.

For successful biofilm formation, attachment of planktonic bacteria to a surface by weak reversible physical forces must be established. If these bacteria are not immediately separated from this surface, they will undergo a phenotypic change that allows for yet stronger binding using adhesins. Once adhered, quorum sensing (cell-to-cell signaling) will facilitate the binding of other bacteria to the infected surface and/or to the initial colonists, thereby forming bacterial colonies. During this period, there is

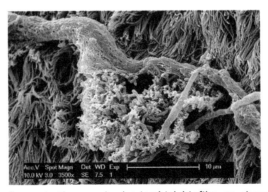

Fig. 1. SEM image demonstrating a mixed microbial biofilm on sinonasal mucosa from a surgical specimen obtained from a patient with chronic rhinosinusitis. Cocci, rods, and hyphae are demonstrated coexisting in the native biofilm. (*Courtesy of* Noam A. Cohen, MD, PhD, and Haibin Yang, MD, University of Pennsylvania, Philadelphia, PA.)

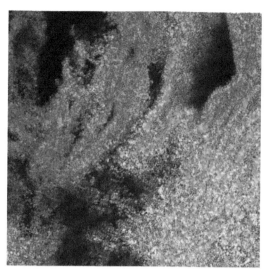

Fig. 2. Mature *Staphylococcus aureus* biofilm grown in the laboratory from clinical isolates. Confocal scanning laser microscopy with BacLite staining (63× magnification).

also formation of the protective glycocalyx, which shrouds the bacteria. Continued growth of the biofilm then occurs by cell division and recruitment. As the cycle continues and the biofilm grows, it matures with the formation of its underlying architecture of microcolonies and channels. Eventually, a dynamic equilibrium is reached by which planktonic bacteria will be present at the biofilm surface, which are then redistributed or seeded through various mechanisms to other areas of the host surface, where further biofilm growth is initiated.

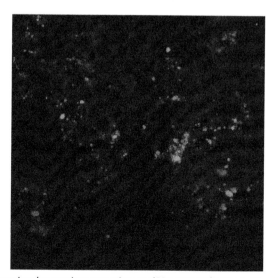

Fig. 3. Confocal scanning laser microscopy image (60× magnification; *Staphylococcus aureus* probe tagged with Alexa 488) demonstrating a *Staphylococcus aureus* bacterial biofilm. (*Courtesy of* Peter John Wormald, MD, and Andrew Foreman, PhD(c), University of Adelaide, Adelaide, Australia.)

Fig. 4. Confocal scanning laser microscopy image (80× magnification; universal fungal probe tagged with Alexa 488) demonstrating a fungal biofilm. (*Courtesy of* Peter John Wormald, MD, and Andrew Foreman, PhD(c), University of Adelaide, Adelaide, Australia.)

Antibiotic Resistance Mechanisms in Biofilms

The recognition of bacterial biofilms was important to explain the recurrence of infection following treatment with antibiotics and the persistence of chronic recalcitrant infections. Bacterial biofilms appear to be able to evade host defenses while also being resistant to current antimicrobial chemotherapeutic agents in concentrations attainable by oral or intravenous administration. Traditional mechanisms of bacterial or fungal resistance to chemotherapeutics by interbacterial transfer of resistance genes contradict the increased bacterial resistance observed in biofilms, but other nonconventional resistance mechanisms such as persister cells that can hide chemotherapeutic target sites likely play an even larger role. As such, biofilm-associated resistance is likely multifactorial and may vary amongst organisms.

The simplest explanation of antibiotic resistance is that biofilms form a physical barrier to antibiotic penetration into the biofilm.[7] However, this may be too simplistic as some antibiotics can perfuse into a biofilm, but there are other mechanisms by which biofilms may limit antimicrobial efficacy.[1,7,8] A consideration is the availability of nutrients and oxygen within the biofilm community. Nutrient and oxygen depletion or waste-product accumulation within the biofilm may lead bacteria to enter a low metabolic state termed the general stress response (GSR). In this reduced metabolic state, secondary to extreme nutrient stress, bacteria become far less susceptible to growth-dependent antimicrobial killing.[2,9] Other considerations include the differentiation of bacterial species into a phenotype resistant to antimicrobials caused by osmotic stress and the resultant down-regulation of transmembrane channels or chemotherapeutic target sites.[7] Efflux pumps or the expression of biofilm-specific antimicrobial resistance genes may also play a role in biofilm persistence.[8] Lastly, quorum sensing may allow for the sharing of genetic information within the bacterial community or the induction and transcription of target genes when signaled.[1] The dispersion of genetic information within the biofilm community minimizes the metabolic cost to individual bacteria, facilitating the persistence of a large number of these genes.

BIOFILMS AND CRS

CRS is a heterogeneous disease with numerous possible causes, which include anatomic factors that lead to ostial obstruction, ciliary dysfunction, bacterial or fungal infection, superantigen stimulation of the immune system, allergy, and immune deficiency. Universal to the pathophysiology of CRS is the persistence of inflammation. The cause of this inflammation in an individual patient is most often indiscernible.

Bacterial involvement in the persistence of CRS has long been suspected; however, the high rate of negative cultures of the sinus cavities in CRS and the absence of a lasting response to antibiotics led specialists to question the role of bacteria in CRS in the late 1990s. Biofilm infection may offer a plausible explanation for the inflammation and observed clinical behavior of CRS. The insurmountable evidence for the presence of biofilm in the setting of chronic infection at various sites throughout the body lends credence to this hypothesis.[6] There exists a similar wealth of information in the literature that supports an important, potentially dominant, role for bacterial biofilms in CRS.

Evidence for Biofilm in CRS

In 2004, the first report supporting the presence of bacterial biofilms in CRS was published.[10] The authors used scanning electron microscopy (SEM) to identify structures consistent with bacterial biofilms present on the biopsied mucosa from a limited number of CRS patients who were clinically nonresponsive to treatment. Confirmation of these findings later came by identifying biofilms on the mucosa of patients with CRS at the time of endoscopic sinus surgery (ESS).[11]

Subsequently, using a rabbit model of sinusitis, investigators were able to show that *Pseudomonas aeruginosa* inoculated in an anatomically obstructed rabbit model of sinusitis could form a biofilm but that no biofilm growth was observed and mucosal histology appeared normal on SEM in the obstructed control sinuses.[12] A recent prospective study in over 150 consecutive CRS patients with mucopurulence identified a nearly 30% rate of bacteria with biofilm-forming capacity as assessed by an in vitro biofilm formation assay.[13] Bacteria identified in this study using conventional culture methods were similar to previous reports; more than 70% of the infections identified were secondary to *Ps aeruginosa* or *Staphylococcus aureus*, or were polymicrobial in nature. A previous study of 38 patients with CRS undergoing ESS detected bacterial biofilm in 44% of the patients using CSLM.[14] None were present in the 9 control patients. The biofilm stain used in this study did not allow for the identification of the organisms involved.

The pathogenic bacteria most commonly implicated in CRS have been identified in patients with CRS to exist in the form of a biofilm. In numerous studies of the bacteriology of CRS done with conventional culture methods, *Staphylococcus aureus* has been identified as one of the most common bacteria to colonize the paranasal sinuses in both asymptomatic postoperative and operative patients with CRS.[15,16] Recently, the use of molecular techniques to identify pathogens in operated patients with CRS has confirmed the presence of *Staphylococcus aureus* in more than 50% of individuals.[17] Similarly, this organism has been demonstrated to occur in the form of a biofilm in patients with CRS, as have coagulase-negative staphylococcus (CNS), *Ps aeruginosa* and *Haemophilus influenzae*.[18–21] The mechanisms by which a *Staphylococcus aureus* biofilm can maintain the inflammation present in CRS remain to be ascertained.

A recent publication used CSLM with fluorescent in situ hybridization and specific molecular probes allowing for identification of *Streptococcus pneumoniae,*

H influenzae, Staphylococcus aureus, and *Ps aeruginosa* to assess mucosal biopsies from individuals undergoing ESS for CRS.[21] Bacterial biofilm was identified in 14 of 18 CRS patients and in 2 of 5 controls. Surprisingly, the principal pathogen identified was *H influenzae,* a respiratory pathogen previously not believed to play a role in CRS. However, these results have not yet been replicated by any other group and not even the use of other molecular techniques has led to the identification of *H influenzae* in other CRS patients, thereby drawing into question the significance of these findings.[17]

These studies demonstrate that biofilms are present in patients with CRS and that they can be identified directly or indirectly in at least one-third of CRS patients with the current technology. In addition, they also suggest that the bacteriology of these bacterial biofilms may not differ radically from what has been described previously for conventional cultures, although this question is not yet fully answered. Together they suggest at least that bacterial biofilms may contribute to the presence of inflammation and the concordant poor response to medical treatment for certain patients with CRS. It remains to be clarified which organisms are primarily involved and the exact mechanisms by which a biofilm may contribute to the inflammation present in CRS. In the absence of an overarching hypothesis linking bacteria at the epithelial surface with the changes in the inner environment, bacterial and host factors need to be considered separately.

Importance of Biofilms in CRS: Bacterial Factors

Although the presence of bacterial biofilms in most patients with CRS is now clearly documented in the literature, their role in the development and persistence of the disease is only beginning to be established. Only two studies have explored the functional importance of biofilms in CRS.

The first study explored the biofilm-forming capacity of bacterial strains recovered from patients with CRS at least 1 year post-ESS.[22] Isolates for *Staphylococcus aureus, Ps aeruginosa,* and CNS were obtained from unselected individuals following ESS. Using an in vitro technique, crystal violet was used to semi-quantitatively determine the biofilm-forming capacity of these isolates. Only patients who had a poor evolution postoperatively had in vitro biofilm-producing capacity with *Ps aeruginosa* or *Staphylococcus aureus* organisms. In patients with a favorable postoperative evolution, biofilm-forming capacity was not present in these two species. The presence of a CNS biofilm did not predispose patients to an unfavorable postoperative course. This study strongly suggests that it is the persistence of pathogenic organisms via biofilm-forming capacity, rather than the simple presence of the biofilm itself, that determines the clinical disease course.

The second study assessed the functional impact of the presence of a biofilm in surgical specimens by retrospectively assessing the postoperative outcome of patients with CRS undergoing ESS with and without nasal polyposis. Using CSLM and a nonspecific BacLite stain, which stains biofilm specifically, they identified bacterial biofilms in 20 of 40 (50%) patients. The investigators found that the detection of biofilms on mucosal biopsy was associated with a greater disease severity according to the preoperative radiological score and also worse postoperative symptoms and mucosal outcomes at follow-up.[23]

Importance of Biofilms in CRS: Host Factors

Although the mechanism by which biofilms influence the severity of sinus disease is not yet clear, there is substantial evidence that the presence of certain pathogenic bacteria in the form of a biofilm are involved in the persistence of CRS. The pathophysiology of bacterial biofilms and their interaction with the sinonasal respiratory mucosa in causing the persistence of CRS disease continue to be an important avenue for research and the modulation of biofilms as a potential therapeutic target.

Staphylococcus aureus, a pathogenic organism frequently recovered in individuals with CRS, has been suggested to contribute to the development of disease via superantigen toxin-producing nonspecific T-cell activation. Persistence of colonization or infection with a superantigen-producing strain of *Staphylococcus aureus* may allow continued production of toxin subsequent to the biofilm protecting the bacteria from antimicrobials and normal host defense mechanisms. Additionally, there is some evidence that change of the bacterial phenotype for the planktonic to the biofilm form may be associated with increased toxin secretion. Exotoxin and biofilm formation are regulated by the accessory gene regulator (agr) locus in the *Staphylococcus aureus* quorum-sensing signaling pathway, thereby making this pathway a potential target for therapeutic intervention.[24]

Alteration of mucosal immunity and local defenses may also facilitate bacterial attachment or subsequent biofilm formation. Toll-like receptor-2 (TLR2), an important component of immunity responsible for recognition of Gram-positive bacteria, has been identified as potentially important in the pathogenesis of CRS. Epithelium cultured from patients with early recurrence of disease following surgery has shown a lower expression of TLR2 than control subjects or those patients with favorable postoperative courses.[25] The important interactions between host and bacteria, in primary nasal epithelial cell strains of *Staphylococcus aureus,* have been demonstrated to suppress the innate immune response by down-regulating TLR expression and TLR-mediated signaling.[26]

Other host genetic factors conferring an increased susceptibility to *Staphylococcus aureus* colonization and to the development of CRS are increasing. A pooling-based genome-wide association study of individuals with nasal polyposis identified polymorphisms in 12 different genes associated with recovery of *Staphylococcus aureus*.[27] Polymorphisms in several genes implicated in innate immunity have also been associated with severe chronic sinusitis, suggesting that variability in response of these genes following contact with bacteria at the epithelial surface may influence development of disease.[28–33]

It is hoped that continued work in this evolving area will allow identification of additional mechanisms linking bacteria and mucosal immunity, and further unravel the intricate complexities of host-bacterial interactions, while identifying targets that are readable to therapeutic intervention.

TREATMENT OF BIOFILMS IN CRS

It has been recognized since the discovery of biofilms that infections caused by bacteria in this form are generally resistant to antimicrobial therapy at levels attainable by oral or intravenous administration. Current potential methods of bacterial biofilm eradication include ventilation of the sinus cavity, killing of the pathogenic bacteria, interfering with the quorum sensing of biofilms, and interfering with the biofilm structure mechanically or chemically. Local chemical and mechanical treatments of biofilms for CRS are potentially advantageous given the enhanced access to the sinus mucosa via patent sinus ostia after ESS. Topical therapy may represent an ideal method for the management of biofilms in post-ESS patients. The optimal therapy remains to be determined, but a number of theoretical concepts and in vitro results may help guide research into this area. These can be loosely grouped into (1) antibacterial strategies and (2) biofilm-disrupting strategies.

Antibacterial Strategies

Biofilm disease not eradicated by standard antimicrobial therapy can persist to cause an intense inflammatory response in patients with refractory CRS. Topical treatment with an antimicrobial may be effective in killing the bacteria, although the concentration may need to be adjusted. An in vivo rabbit model of maxillary sinusitis showed that Ps aeruginosa biofilms are not eradicated with topical tobramycin or saline treatments,[34] and that treatment with subtherapeutic levels may actually increase biofilm formation. Another in vitro study using moxifloxacin at levels approaching minimal inhibitory concentrations (MICs) attainable with oral antibiotic therapy had no effect on biofilms grown from clinical isolates of Staphylococcus aureus. Concentrations at 1000 times the MIC of moxifloxacin were required to effect a log 2.0 to 2.5 reduction (or a reduction >99%) in the number of viable bacteria in vitro in a mature Staphylococcus aureus biofilm.[35] Despite bacterial killing, the biofilm matrix persisted and could potentially act as a scaffold for re-infection. This underlines the need to address the bacteria and the biofilm matrix when considering therapy.

Recently, mupirocin has been shown to result in a reduction of biofilm-forming Staphylococcus aureus clinical isolates. Mupirocin was capable of reducing biofilm mass by greater than 90% at concentrations of 125 µg/mL or less in all Staphylococcus aureus isolates, suggesting that topical irrigations with this agent could be a treatment for Staphylococcus aureus biofilm disease.[36] In a small cohort of patients with recalcitrant Staphylococcus aureus culture-positive CRS disease, 0.05% mupirocin was shown to be effective at decreasing patient symptoms and improving endoscopic findings over a 3-week treatment period. Patients were not tested for the presence of biofilm, but a negative culture result was attained in 15 of 16 patients.[37]

An innate immunity protein emanating from the sinonasal mucosa, LL-37-derived antimicrobial peptide, has been tested in an animal model of pseudomonas sinusitis. It was found that this peptide did result in a significant decrease in the infection by this organism after 10 days of irrigation. However, the authors also found that although it was effective as the dose of the antimicrobial peptide increased, the resultant mucosal and bone inflammation and ciliotoxicity also increased.[38]

Lastly, one of the most novel antibacterial agents to have been tested to date is manuka honey, which has been shown in vitro to be an extremely effective agent for the eradication of both Staphylococcus aureus and Ps aeruginosa in planktonic or biofilm forms.[39] Given its effectiveness for the treatment of chronic cutaneous wounds, its effects on normal respiratory mucosa are currently being characterized but are promising given early results while maintaining in vivo efficacy.[40] (Shaun Kilty, MD, Ottawa, Ontario, Canada; June, 2009, personal communication.)

Biofilm-Disrupting Strategies

Much of the evidence for the mechanical treatment of bacterial biofilms originates from orthopedic research. The infection of hip implants is particularly problematic because of the operative and medical treatments that must ensue. Therefore, methods for treating and preventing these biofilm-mediated infections are extremely important.[41]

In some of the first studies, chemical treatments produced a logarithmic reduction in the biofilm load of Staphylococcus species and Ps aeruginosa on implant devices. This was then improved by the addition of a mechanical pressure irrigation system.[42] Tests on in vivo models were then used to show that some chemicals, when used with mechanical irrigation, can have a greater impact on infections caused by one organism but not others. Castile soap, for example, demonstrated better efficacy for the treatment of Ps aeruginosa infection, whereas benzalkonium chloride had a greater effect on wounds containing *Staphylococcus aureus*.[43] Generally, the use of a surfactant solution rather than antibiotic or saline has been shown to have a greater efficacy in treating these infections in an orthopedic model because they work by disrupting the bonds of the organism to the infected (usually artificial) surface.[44]

As an example of a simple biofilm-disrupting strategy, baby shampoo, a nonionic surfactant, has been used in patients with CRS and evidence of recalcitrant disease following sinus surgery. Again in a small cohort, a 1% solution was used for sinonasal irrigations twice daily for 4 weeks. More than 10% of patients could not complete the study because of treatment side effects; overall the greatest improvement was in the subjective patient rating of postnasal drip and thickened mucus. These results suggest that further development of surfactant-based therapies may be of interest.[45]

To maximize the effect of disruption strategies, it has been suggested to develop an irrigation device that creates a shear force while delivering a nontoxic, water-soluble, low-viscosity surfactant. A pressure irrigation system using a mixture of sterile water, citric acid, and caprylyl sulfobetaine (zwitterionic surfactant) (CAZS) has been assessed in vitro to evaluate its effectiveness at reducing the biomass of human sinus bacterial biofilms.[46] When tested on the biofilm mass of *Staphylococcus aureus* and *Ps aeruginosa*, the use of saline irrigation alone produced a 2-log reduction in colony-forming units (CFU), whereas CAZS with high-pressure irrigation produced a synergistic effect, with 3.9-log (*Staphylococcus aureus*) and 5.2-log (*Ps aeruginosa*) reductions in CFU. However, application of this substance to mucosal cells in animal models led to ciliary shedding at the level of the epithelium, with increased bacterial adhesion noted during the maximal phase of damage. This underlines the importance of verifying in vitro results in appropriate models before their use in the clinical setting.

Mupirocin and CAZS pressure irrigation have been tested in vivo using a sheep animal model of frontal chronic sinusitis. *Staphylococcus aureus* biofilms in the frontal sinuses were treated with these topical agents alone or together. CSLM was used to confirm the presence or absence of biofilms and the extent of biofilm reduction was quantified using fluorescent in situ hybridization and CFU counts. Treatment with mupirocin produced the greatest reduction in biofilm surface area coverage in comparison with the CAZS solution and all other topical treatments that were trialed. Mupirocin irrigation over a 5-day treatment period demonstrated a clear advantage over CAZS at the end of the 8-day trial period.[47]

In summary, to date there have been some encouraging results for trials of topical therapies in the treatment of biofilm-associated CRS. The ideal topical treatment still remains to be developed. The ideal therapy will combine bactericidal effects with a means for reducing the biofilm mass. This may require combining chemical with mechanical strategies. Several different treatments may emerge over time for this purpose, each with its own target of preference. For this to occur, rapid noninvasive methods for the in vivo detection of biofilm need to be developed.

SUMMARY

The detection of bacterial biofilms in the upper respiratory tract has been a significant development in understanding the pathophysiology of CRS. It is possible that biofilm disease has the central role in dictating the clinical manifestations of the disease while also accounting for its recurrent nature. Although the exact mechanism by which this form of infection causes persistent mucosal inflammation is yet to be understood, future directions for investigation in CRS will include the development of rapid clinical tests that facilitate the diagnosis of infection by a bacterial biofilm. Similarly, the eradication or control of these infections will depend upon the production of efficacious topical treatments and even the manipulation of quorum-sensing behavior. Given the potential toxicity of topical therapies to the sinus epithelium, it is important that agents are assessed in cellular and animal models for toxicity before their use in humans.

REFERENCES

1. Donlan RM, Costerton JW. Biofilms: survival mechanisms of clinically relevant microorganisms. Clin Microbiol Rev 2002;15(2):167–93.
2. Costerton JW, Geesey GG, Cheng GK. How bacteria stick. Sci Am 1978;238(1):86–95.
3. Davies DG, Parsek MR, Pearson JP, et al. The involvement of cell-to-cell signals in the development of a bacterial biofilm. Science 1998;280(5361):295–8.
4. Manning SC. Basics of biofilm in clinical otolaryngology. Ear Nose Throat J 2003;82(8 Suppl 2):18–20.
5. Chole RA, Faddis BT. Evidence for microbial biofilms in cholesteatomas. Arch Otolaryngol Head Neck Surg 2002;128(10):1129–33.
6. Costerton W, Veeh R, Shirtliff M, et al. The application of biofilm science to the study and control of chronic bacterial infections. J Clin Invest 2003;112(10):1466–77.
7. Stewart PS, Costerton JW. Antibiotic resistance of bacteria in biofilms. Lancet 2001;358(9276):135–8.
8. Patel R. Biofilms and antimicrobial resistance. Clin Orthop Relat Res 2005;437:41–7.
9. Costerton JW, Stewart PS, Greenberg EP. Bacterial biofilms: a common cause of persistent infections. Science 1999;284(5418):1318–22.
10. Cryer J, Shipor I, Perloff JR, et al. Evidence of bacterial biofilms in human chronic sinusitis. ORL J Otorhinolaryngol Relat Spec 2004;66(3):155–8.
11. Ramadan HH, Sanclement JA, Thomas JG. Chronic rhinosinusitis and biofilms. Otolaryngol Head Neck Surg 2005;132(3):414–7.
12. Perloff JR, Palmer JN. Evidence of bacterial biofilms in a rabbit model of sinusitis. Am J Rhinol 2005;19(1):1–6.
13. Prince AA, Steiger JD, Khalid AN, et al. Prevalence of biofilm-forming bacteria in chronic rhinosinusitis. Am J Rhinol 2008;22:239–45.
14. Psaltis AJ, Ha KR, Beule AG, et al. Confocal scanning laser microscopy evidence of biofilms in patients with chronic rhinosinusitis. Laryngoscope 2007;117(7):1302–6.
15. Desrosiers M, Hussain A, Frenkiel S, et al. Intranasal corticosteroid use is associated with lower rates of bacterial recovery in chronic rhinosinusitis. Otolaryngol Head Neck Surg 2007;136(4):605–9.
16. Al-Shemari H, Abou-Hamad W, Libman M, et al. Bacteriology of the sinus cavities of asymptomatic individuals after endoscopic sinus surgery. J Otolaryngol 2007;36(1):43–8.
17. Stephenson M-F, Mfuna Endam L, Dowd S et al. Molecular characterization of the polymicrobial flora in chronic rhinosinusitis. J Otolaryngol Head Neck Surg, in press.
18. Sanclement JA, Webster P, Thomas J, et al. Bacterial biofilms in surgical specimens of patients with chronic rhinosinusitis. Laryngoscope 2005;115(4):578–82.
19. Ferguson BJ, Stolz DB. Demonstration of biofilm in human bacterial chronic rhinosinusitis. Am J Rhinol 2005;19(5):452–7.

20. Bendouah Z, Barbeau J, Hamad WA, et al. Use of an in vitro assay for determination of biofilm-forming capacity of bacteria in chronic rhinosinusitis. Am J Rhinol 2006;20(5):434–8.
21. Sanderson SR, Leid JG, Hunsaker DH. Bacterial biofilms on the sinus mucosa of human subjects with chronic rhinosinusitis. Laryngoscope 2006;116(7):1121–6.
22. Bendouah Z, Barbeau J, Hamad WA, et al. Biofilm formation by *Staphylococcus aureus* and *Pseudomonas aeruginosa* is associated with an unfavorable evolution after surgery for chronic sinusitis and nasal polyposis. Otolaryngol Head Neck Surg 2006;134(6):991–6.
23. Psaltis AJ, Weitzel EK, Ha KR, Wormald PJ. The effect of bacterial biofilms and post-sinus surgical outcomes. Am J Rhinol 2008;22(1):1–6.
24. Iwatsuki K, Yamasaki O, Morizane S, et al. Staphylococcal cutaneous infections: invasion, evasion and aggression. J Dermatol Sci 2006;42:203–14.
25. Lane AP, Truong-Tran QA, Schleimer RP. Altered expression of genes associated with innate immunity and inflammation in recalcitrant rhinosinusitis with polyps. Am J Rhinol 2006;20:138–44.
26. Sivaraman K, Venkataraman N, Tsai J, et al. Genome sequencing and analysis reveals possible determinants of *Staphylococcus aureus* nasal carriage. BMC Genomics 2008;9:433–4.
27. Cormier C, Mfuna Endam L, Bossé Y, et al. Genes conferring susceptibility to *Staphylococcus aureus* colonisation in patients with chronic rhinosinusitis with nasal polyposis. Presented at The 63rd Annual Meeting of the Canadian Society of Otolaryngology-Head and Neck Surgery, May 10–13, 2009, Halifax, Nova Scotia, Canada.
28. Cormier C, Bossé Y, Mfuna Endam L, et al. Polymorphisms in the tumour necrosis factor alpha-induced protein 3 (TNFAIP3) gene are associated with chronic rhinosinusitis. J Otolaryngol Head Neck Surg 2009;38(1):133–41.
29. Tewfik M, Bossé Y, Hudson T, et al. Total serum IgE is related to polymorphisms in IRAK-4 in a population with chronic rhinosinustis. Allergy 2009;64(5):746–53.
30. Bossé Y, Bacot F, Montpetit A, et al. Identification of susceptibility genes for complex diseases using pooling-based genome-wide association scans. Hum Genet 2009;125(3):305–18.
31. Mfuna Endam L, Bossé Y, Filali-Mouhim A, et al. Polymorphisms in the interleukin 22 receptor alpha-1 gene are associated with severe chronic rhinosinusitis. Otolaryngol Head Neck Surg 2009;140(5):741–7.
32. Castano R, Bossé Y, Mfuna Endam L, et al. Evidence of association of Interleukin 1 receptor-like 1 gene polymorphisms with surgery unresponsive chronic rhinosinusitis. Am J Rhinol Allergy 2009;23:977–84.
33. Kilty SJ, Bossé Y, Cormier C et al. Polymorphisms in the SERPINA1 gene are associated with severe chronic rhinosinusitis unresponsive to medical therapy. Am J Rhinol Allergy, in press.
34. Chiu AG, Antunes MB, Palmer JN, et al. Evaluation of the in vivo efficacy of topical tobramycin against pseudomonas sinonasal biofilms. J Antimicrob Chemother 2007;59(6):1130–4.
35. Desrosiers M, Bendouah Z, Barbeau J. Effectiveness of topical antibiotics on *Staphylococcus aureus* in vitro. Am J Rhinol 2007;21(2):149–53.
36. Ha KR, Psaltis AJ, Butcher AR, et al. In vitro activity of mupirocin on clinical isolates of *Staphylococcus aureus* and its potential implications in chronic rhinosinusitis. Laryngoscope 2008;118(3):535–40.
37. Uren B, Psaltis A, Wormald PJ. Nasal lavage with mupirocin for the treatment of surgically recalcitrant chronic rhinosinusitis. Laryngoscope 2008;118:1677–80.

38. Chennupati SK, Chiu AG, Tamashiro E, et al. Effects of an LL-37-derived antimicrobial peptide in an animal model of biofilm Pseudomonas sinusitis. Am J Rhinol Allergy 2009;23(1):46–51.
39. Alandejani T, Marsan J, Ferris W, et al. Effectiveness of honey on *Staphylococcus aureus* and *Pseudomonas aeruginosa* biofilms. Otolaryngol Head Neck Surg 2009;141(1):114–8.
40. Merckoll P, Jonassen TØ, Vad ME, et al. Bacteria, biofilm and honey: a study of the effects of honey on 'planktonic' and biofilm-embedded chronic wound bacteria. Scand J Infect Dis 2009;41(5):341–7.
41. Canadian Institute for Health Information (CIHI). Canadian Joint Replacement Registry (CJRR) Bulletin: surgical and orthopaedic implant information for total hip and total knee replacement procedures performed in Canada, May 2001–March 2002. Toronto (ON): CIHI; 2002.
42. Moussa FW, Gainor BJ, Anglen JO, et al. Disinfecting agents for removing adherent bacteria from orthopaedic hardware. Clin Orthop Relat Res 1996;329:255–62.
43. Conroy BP, Anglen JO, Simpson WA, et al. Comparison of castile soap, benzalkonium chloride, and bacitracin as irrigation solutions for complex contaminated orthopaedic wounds. J Orthop Trauma 1999;13(5):332–7.
44. Anglen JO, Gainor BJ, Simpson WA, et al. The use of detergent irrigation for musculoskeletal wounds. Int Orthop 2003;27(1):40–6.
45. Chiu AG, Palmer JN, Woodworth BA, et al. Baby shampoo nasal irrigations for the symptomatic post-functional endoscopic sinus surgery patient. Am J Rhinol 2008;22:34–7.
46. Desrosiers M, Myntti M, James G. Methods for removing bacterial biofilms: in vitro study using clinical chronic rhinosinusitis specimens. Am J Rhinol 2007;21(5):527–32.
47. Le T, Psaltis A, Tan LW, et al. The efficacy of topical antibiofilm agents in a sheep model of rhinosinusitis. Am J Rhinol 2008;22:560–7.

Corticosteroid Treatment in Chronic Rhinosinusitis: The Possibilities and the Limits

Joaquim Mullol, MD, PhD[a,b],*, Andrés Obando, MD[a,1], Laura Pujols, PhD[b], Isam Alobid, MD, PhD[a]

KEYWORDS

- Corticosteroids • Chronic rhinosinusitis • Nasal polyps
- Endoscopic sinus surgery • Efficay and safety

Chronic rhinosinusitis (CRS), with (CRwNP) and without (CRsNP) nasal polyps, is one of the most frequent chronic inflammatory diseases, with inflammation of the nasal and paranasal sinus mucosa and sinonasal symptoms lasting for more than 12 consecutive weeks.[1] The treatment of CRS has been considered as a major subject in various studies resulting from respective consensus groups and task forces in the United States[2] and Europe.[3] In CRwNP and CRsNP, medical treatment, including nasal and

Financial disclosure: J.M. is or has been a member of National or International Scientific Advisory Boards for UCB Pharchim, Grupo Uriach SA, Schering-Plough, GSK, Hartington Pharmaceuticals, MSD, and FAES. He has received grants for research projects from Schering-Plough, Grupo Uriach SA, UCB Pharchim, and MSD; and has been national or/and international coordinator or main investigator of clinical trials for UCB Farma, FAES, Grupo Uriach SA, and Schering-Plough. I.A. has received grants for research projects from Schering-Plough, Grupo Uriach, and MSD; and has been investigator collaborator of clinical trials for Grupo Uriach SA and Schering-Plough. A.O. and L.P. have no conflicts of interest or financial disclosure. Funding: The research group is sponsored in part by *Generalitat de Catalunya, Centro de Investigaciones Biomédicas en Red de Enfermedades Respiratorias* (CIBERES) and Global Allergy and Asthma European Network (GA²LEN). L.P. is a FIS investigator from *Instituto Carlos III - Fondo de Investigación Sanitaria*. A.O. was awarded a grant from *Centro de Desarrollo Estratégico e Información en Salud y Seguridad Social, Caja Costaricense del Seguro Social* (CENDEISSS, Costa Rica).

[1]Address after October 1, 2009: Ofi.Centauro, Oficina 320, Guadalupe, San José, Costa Rica.
[a] Unitat de Rinologia & Clínica de l'Olfacte, Department of Otorhinolaryngology, Hospital Clínic, c/Villarroel, 170 Barcelona 08036, Catalonia, Spain
[b] Clinical and Experimental Respiratory Immunoallergy, Institut d'Investigacions Biomèdiques August Pi i Sunyer (IDIBAPS), c/Villarroel 170, Barcelona 08036, Catalonia, Spain
* Corresponding author. Unitat de Rinologia & Clínica de l'Olfacte, Department of Otorhinolaryngology, Hospital Clínic, c/Villarroel, 170 Barcelona 08036, Catalonia, Spain.
E-mail address: jmullol@clinic.ub.es (J. Mullol).

Immunol Allergy Clin N Am 29 (2009) 657–668
doi:10.1016/j.iac.2009.07.001
0889-8561/09/$ – see front matter © 2009 Elsevier Inc. All rights reserved.

oral corticosteroids, constitutes the first step in therapy. Corticosteroids are the mainstay of treatment and are the most effective drugs for treating airway inflammatory diseases, such as asthma,[4] allergic rhinitis,[5,6] and CRS.[3] Endoscopic sinus surgery is recommended only when medical treatment fails. This article reviews the steroid mechanism of action as well as the efficacy, safety, and therapeutic recommendations for the use of corticosteroids in the treatment of CRS, including nasal polyps.

MECHANISM OF ACTION OF CORTICOSTEROIDS

The clinical efficacy of corticosteroids is achieved by a combination of anti-inflammatory effects such as reducing proinflammatory or increasing anti-inflammatory gene transcription, along with their ability to reduce airway inflammatory cell infiltration, including eosinophils, T lymphocytes, mast cells, and dendritic cells, and to suppress the production of proinflammatory mediators, cell chemotactic factors, and adhesion molecules.

The predominant effect of corticosteroids is to switch off a variety of inflammatory protein-encoding genes (cytokines, chemokines, adhesion molecules, inflammatory enzymes, receptors, and other proteins) that have been activated during the chronic inflammatory process. These effects are exerted by intracellular activation of the glucocorticoid receptor (GR).[7,8]

In its inactive state, the GR exists as a cytosolic protein bound to 2 heat-shock protein 90 chaperonin molecules. Binding to the corticosteroid ligand results in a conformational change that allows disassociation of the GR from the protein complex. As homodimer, the activated ligand-bound GR translocates into the nucleus where it binds at specific sequences in the DNA promoter region of corticosteroid response genes, known as glucocorticoid response elements (GREs), leading to changes in gene transcription. This interaction classically reduces proinflammatory or increases anti-inflammatory gene transcription (transactivation) (**Fig. 1**). As monodimer, GR can also regulate gene expression through direct interaction with transcription factors (transrepression) such as activator protein 1 (AP-1) and nuclear factor-κB (NF-κB).[9,10] These transcription factors are responsible for the increased expression of a variety of inflammatory proteins during inflammation. Thus, the activated GR inhibits the proinflammatory effects of a variety of cytokines and other inflammatory molecules through its interaction with these transcription factors.[11]

Two human isoforms of GR have been identified as GRα and GRβ. GRα has a widespread distribution in cells and tissues[12] and, with the participation of numerous cofactors, is responsible for the induction and repression of target genes.[7] GRβ acts as a dominant negative inhibitor of GRα-mediated transactivation and transrepression.[13] However, although it is expressed in numerous cells and tissues, GRβ has a very low level of expression compared with GRα.[12]

Increased expression of GRβ has been reported in different inflammatory diseases (eg, bronchial asthma, ulcerative colitis, and nasal polyposis), and has been proposed as one of the potential mechanisms explaining glucocorticoid resistance.[14] The expression of GRβ is higher in nasal polyps than in nasal mucosa epithelial cells, and is correlated with increased infiltration of inflammatory cells.[15] Although downregulation of GRα after treatment with glucocorticoids has been reported[16] and could account for secondary steroid resistance, a recent study in patients with nasal polyps has shown that this effect does not occur in vivo.[17]

PHARMACOLOGY OF CORTICOSTEROIDS

Quantification of GR binding affinity is one of the methods used to measure glucocorticoid potency. The highest relative receptor affinity is associated with some of the

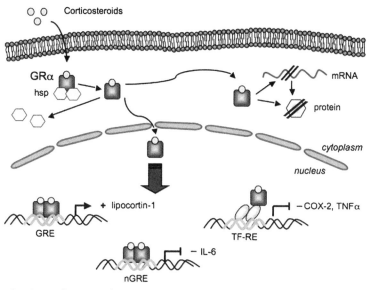

Fig. 1. Mechanisms of action of corticosteroids. After passing the cell membrane by passive diffusion, corticosteroids bind to glucocorticoid receptor α (GRα), associated heat-shock proteins (hsp) are released, and the ligand-bound receptor translocates into the nucleus. A GRα-dimer can bind glucocorticoid response elements (GRE) on the promoter region of target genes and activate gene transcription. Binding of GRα to a negative GRE (nGRE) leads to repression. Protein-protein interactions between GRα and transcription factors, such as nuclear factor-κB and activator protein-1, repress the transcription of proinflammatory genes (transrepression) such as cyclooxygenase-2 (COX-2) or tumor necrosis factor-α (TNFα). GRα can alter the mRNA or protein stability of inflammatory mediators. IL, interleukin; TF-RE, transcription factor-response element. (*Data from* Refs.[12–17])

newest compounds such as fluticasone furoate, mometasone furoate, and fluticasone propionate, and the poorest receptor affinity is related to dexamethasone (**Table 1**).[18] However, of importance is that there is no evidence of a linear association between glucocorticoid potency and clinical response, meaning that there is no evidence that a higher receptor affinity correlates with a superior clinical efficacy.[19]

There are important pharmacokinetic properties that determine the concentration and disposition of intranasal steroids at the receptor site and the potential for the drug to reach the systemic circulation. The more lipophilic the compounds, the faster they are absorbed by the nasal mucosa, the longer they are retained in nasal tissue which increases exposure to the GR,[20] and the higher is their binding to plasma proteins. This characteristic may be attributed to the accumulation of drug in other tissues and contribute to unwanted side effects.[19] The order of lipid solubility for corticosteroids has been reported as: mometasone furoate > fluticasone propionate > beclometasone dipropionate > budesonide > triamcinolone acetonide > flunisolide.[20]

In addition, up to 50% of systemic bioavailability of an intranasal steroid is also dependent on the direct systemic absorption rate through nasal tissue (see **Table 1**).[21] This process occurs to bypass the protective hepatic first-pass mechanism, which is higher among older compounds such as flunisolide, beclomethasone, and budesonide. Fluticasone propionate and mometasone furoate have an extensive first-pass hepatic metabolism due to their absorption from the gastrointestinal tract, which avoids their

Table 1
Relative receptor affinity (RRA) and bioavailability of intranasal corticosteroids

Corticosteroid	RRA[a]	Bioavailability (%)
Fluticasone furoate	2,989	0.5
Mometasone furoate	2,244	< 0.1
Fluticasone propionate	1,775	0.51 (spray) 0.06 (nasal drops)
Beclomethasone dipropionate	1,345	44
Ciclesonide AP	1,212	< 0.1
Budesonide	855	31
Triamcinolone	233	44
Flunisolide	177	40–50
Dexamethasone	100	> 80

[a] RRA compared with dexamethasone (100).
Data from Derendorf H, Meltzer EO. Molecular and clinical pharmacology of intranasal corticosteroids: clinical and therapeutic implications. Allergy 2008;63(10):1292–300.

systemic absorption,[22] whereas fluticasone furoate has been reported as having a very high binding affinity to nasal tissue[18] and hence, a low systemic absorption.

EFFICACY AND SAFETY OF CORTICOSTEROIDS
Intranasal Corticosteroids

Efficacy
The introduction of topically administered corticosteroid has improved the treatment of upper and lower airway inflammatory diseases. Since 1975 several placebo-controlled studies have reported the benefit of treating CRwNP patients with intranasal corticosteroids. Nowadays, there is a high level of evidence (Ia) demonstrating their positive effect on the reduction of polyp size, reflected in the improvement of nasal cavity volume measured with acoustic rhinometry,[23] as well as on nasal symptoms,[3] including nasal congestion, sneezing, rhinorrea, loss of smell, and postnasal drip.[24–27] Some studies in nasal polyp patients have reported no decrease in polyp size together with a significant improvement of nasal symptoms.[28–30]

Even though symptoms like nasal blockage and rhinorrea respond well to topical nasal steroids, controversial findings on the improvement of the sense of smell have been reported.[27,31] The sense of smell constitutes an important warning system for gas leaking, smoke, food spoilage, or air pollution. CRS with and without polyps is a major cause of smell loss, causing an important impact on quality of life (QoL) and constituting an especially troublesome symptom in the elderly, with association of loss of appetite and weight, and the onset of depression.[32] Nasal drops have been shown to be more effective than nasal spray in improving the sense of smell in CRwNP.[33]

In relation to smell disorders, CRwNP has a considerable impact on QoL, especially on the mental health component compared with the physical health component. Two different studies have demonstrated that corticosteroids improve QoL especially in body pain, general health, vitality, social functioning, and mental health domains.[32,34] Both medical (combination of oral and intranasal steroids) and surgical (endoscopic sinus surgery followed by intranasal steroids) treatments led to similar long-term improvement of QoL.[32]

CRwNP patients with persistent symptoms who do not satisfactorily respond to long-term topical intranasal and to short-term oral corticosteroid treatment may benefit from endoscopic sinus surgery (ESS).[3] The use of intranasal corticosteroids in the postoperative period has shown an improvement in nasal symptoms, a reduction in the need for oral corticoids rescue courses, and a reduced recurrence rate of nasal polyps.[35,36]

The role of topical corticosteroids in CRsNP has been less extensively studied. There are 5 randomized control trials investigating the use of topical corticosteroids in CRsNP.[37–41] Two of these trials involved intrasinus installation of the drug, whereas the other 3 involved topical treatment. Four of the 5 trials demonstrated a significant improvement in symptoms, whereas none demonstrated an increase in the infection rate.

Safety

Although nasal topical corticosteroids are very safe in general, they are not completely devoid of systemic and local side effects. Several factors such as molecular characteristics of corticosteroids, dose prescription, mode of delivery, and severity of the underlying disease may influence steroid absorption into systemic circulation.[42] Systemic bioavailability of intranasal corticosteroids varies from less than 1% for some new molecules (mometasone, fluticasone) to up to 40% to 50% for older molecules (budesonide, triamcinolone), which may influence the risk of systemic adverse effects.[43] There is no clear evidence that the use of nasal corticosteroids at recommended doses correlates with systemic changes in bone mineral biology, cataracts, or glaucoma. In a matched nested case-control analysis performed in a population-based cohort of elderly people, the use of nasal corticosteroids was not associated with an increased risk of cataracts that required extraction.[44] At recommended doses, adrenal suppression may occur with some nasal corticosteroids but the clinical relevance remains uncertain, whereas the overuse of nasal corticosteroids may be responsible for adrenal insufficiency and decrease in bone mineral density.[45] Extensive studies have not identified significant effects on the hypothalamic-pituitary-adrenal (HPA) axis with continued treatment.[46] A unique study has reported a small effect on the growth of children receiving a standard dosage of beclomethasone over 1 year of treatment.[47] However, this effect has not been found in prospective studies using intranasal corticosteroids with low systemic bioavailability.[48]

In addition, nasal biopsy studies have not shown any detrimental structural effects within the nasal mucosa with long-term administration of intranasal corticosteroids.[43] Minor nose bleeding associated with corticosteroid use, present in a small proportion of the patients, has been attributed to a vasoconstrictor activity of the steroid molecules.[49] In summary, special care has to be taken especially in selected populations such as children, and in patients with comorbid conditions such as asthma, in whom the overall steroid intake may be high due to the administration of both intranasal and inhaled corticosteroid.[42]

Oral Corticosteroids

Efficacy

Systemic steroids are reserved for refractory cases or when a relatively rapid short-term improvement is needed. The clinical effects of oral corticosteroids in CRwNP and CRsNP have been documented to a lesser extent than those of intranasal steroids. Nevertheless, several studies in CRwNP have reported a rapid symptomatic improvement, particularly in nasal obstruction and smell,[50] also achieving a significant polyp size reduction as well as a reduction of imaging (computed tomography, magnetic resonance imaging) changes when prednisone is being given orally for 2 weeks.[27,51] A usual initial dose in adults would be prednisone at 0.5 to 1 mg/kg/d with a tapered reduction of 5 to 10 mg every 2 to 3 days over a period of 2 to 3 weeks.[27] In CRsNP patients, although a similar treatment protocol may be recommended, there are no data showing efficacy of oral corticosteroids, either before or after surgery.[3]

Safety

The anti-inflammatory effects of oral steroids cannot be separated from their metabolic effects. Suppression of the HPA axis, osteoporosis or changes in bone mineral density, growth retardation in children, and cataracts and glaucoma have been reported as the main adverse effects of corticosteroid oral treatment. Short courses of oral corticosteroids are effective and safe in CRwNP,[3] but a repeated or prolonged use of oral steroids may be associated with an enhanced risk of systemic side effects.[52]

Depot Injection or Local Injection of Corticosteroids

There are no good randomized studies on steroid depot injection. The injection of local corticosteroids into the inferior turbinate has recently been associated with a significantly lower rate of complications than surgical excision of nasal polyps and with a reduced need for further surgical intervention.[53] However, the reports of fat necrosis at the site of the injection and blindness following endonasal injection have demonstrated that this treatment is not recommendable.[54]

SPECIAL CONSIDERATIONS AND LIMITS
Corticosteroids in Children with Chronic Rhinosinusitis

Data on steroid treatment of CRS in children are limited, with no studies on the efficacy of topical corticosteroids in pediatric CRS. However, there are many studies showing that local corticosteroids are effective and safe in children with rhinitis.[55–57] Safety aspects of intranasal steroids in children have been reviewed in several reports,[58] especially those side effects related to bone growth and height. Studies based on knemometry, considered the most reliable and sensitive indicator, have shown different and controversial results. An early study reported a slower leg growth velocity among children receiving high-dose intranasal budesonide for 6 weeks compared with a pretreatment run-in period,[59] whereas other studies using budesonide, mometasone furoate, and fluticasone propionate have not demonstrated significant changes in leg growth velocity.[60,61] Using stadiometry, a mechanical method used to measure height, the evaluation of similar steroid molecules did not report any significant negative effects on height.[47,62–64] Among studies based on stadiometry, only one has reported a small mean increase in height among children treated with high-dose intranasal beclomethasone for 1 year compared with placebo.[65]

Corticosteroids in Pregnant Chronic Rhinosinusitis Patients

Concerning their use in pregnancy, the US Food and Drug Administration has classified intranasal steroids as category C, except for budesonide, whose classification has been upgraded to category B in early pregnancy.[66] Studies on the use of intranasal corticosteroid in pregnancy are limited in number, whereas no studies on pregnant CRS patients have been conducted. Nevertheless, the use of inhaled steroids has been studied in asthmatic pregnant women; the results showed that beclomethasone and triamcinolone were not associated with preeclampsia, preterm weight, and low birth weight.[66,67] In pregnant women with rhinitis, the use of fluticasone propionate

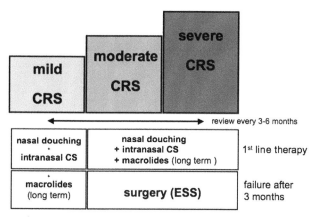

Fig. 2. Indication of corticosteroids in the management scheme of adult patients with CRS without nasal polyps, based on the EP³OS consensus. (*Data from* Fokkens W, Lund V, Mullol J, et al. EP³OS 2007: European position paper on rhinosinusitis and nasal polyps 2007. Rhinology 2007;20:1–136.)

for 8 weeks after the first trimester did not show any significant effect on maternal cortisol, or any difference in ultrasound measures of fetal growth or pregnancy outcome.[68]

There are no documented epidemiologic studies with data on use of the newer intranasal steroids (fluticasone propionate, mometasone furoate) during pregnancy. Inhaled steroids have not been associated with an increase in congenital malformations in humans, and it could be assumed that a similar finding would be true for intranasal steroids in pregnant CRS patients (level of evidence IV).

The use of oral corticosteroids during the first trimester should be restricted to life-threatening conditions. Although no study has associated the use of oral steroids with a major teratogenic risk and the presence of major congenital malformations, an increased association with oral clefts has been reported.[69] Oral corticosteroids have been associated with the occurrence of preeclampsia in asthmatic pregnant women, but this association could also be due to common pathogenic factors shared by patients with severe asthma and those experiencing preeclampsia.[70,71]

Table 2
Levels of evidence and recommendations for corticosteroids in CRS patients, with and without nasal polyps

	Intranasal Corticosteroids		Oral Corticosteroids	
	Evidence Level	Recommendation	Evidence Level	Recommendation
CRS without nasal polyps				
Preoperative	Ib	A	No data	D
Postoperative	Ib	B	No data	D
CRS with nasal polyps				
Preoperative	Ib	A	Ib	A
Postoperative	Ib	A	III	C

Abbreviation: CRS, chronic rhinosinusitis.
Data from Fokkens W, Lund V, Mullol J, et al. EP³OS 2007: European position paper on rhinosinusitis and nasal polyps 2007. Rhinology 2007;20:1–136.

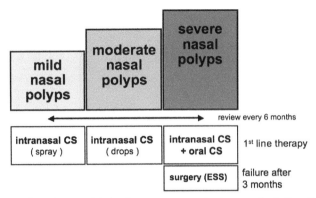

Fig. 3. Indication of corticosteroids in the management scheme of adult patients with CRS with nasal polyps, based on the EP³OS consensus. (*Data from* Fokkens W, Lund V, Mullol J, et al. EP³OS 2007: European position paper on rhinosinusitis and nasal polyps 2007. Rhinology 2007;20:1–136.)

CORTICOSTEROID RECOMMENDATIONS IN CHRONIC RHINOSINUSITIS

The American Rhinosinusitis Initiative[72] and the European EPO³S guidelines[3] on CRS have clinically defined CRS as the presence of nasal congestion/blockage in combination with nasal discharge, $\pm$ facial pain/pressure, $\pm$ reduction or loss of smell lasting for more than 12 weeks, with either: endoscopic signs of nasal polyps and/or mucopurulent discharge, and/or edema/mucosal obstruction in middle meatus, and/or computed tomography changes within the ostiomeatal complex and/or sinuses. The severity of CRS including nasal polyps may be estimated and classified using a visual analog score (VAS) in mild (VAS ≤ 3), moderate (VAS >3–7), and severe (VAS >7–10).

According to the EP³OS consensus, there are evidence-based recommendations for using corticosteroids in CRS. In CRsNP, topical steroids are recommended as the first line of therapy in patients with mild to moderate/severe disease as well as in the follow-up period (**Fig. 2** and **Table 2**), with high level of evidence (Ib) and recommendation (A). Related to oral corticosteroids, there are insufficient efficacy data allowing their recommendation in CRsNP.

In CRwNP, the use of topical intranasal corticosteroids has a high evidence level (Ib) and recommendation (A). Nasal spray is recommended for the mild disease whereas corticosteroid drops are recommended for the moderate disease (**Fig. 3** and **Table 2**). A recent meta-analysis concluded that intranasal corticosteroids have a positive effect, providing significant improvement in polyp size compared with controls.[73] Long-term treatment with intranasal corticosteroids is recommended in patients with a mild to severe disease both before surgery and having undergone surgery. The use of systemic steroids in CRwNP also has a high level of evidence (Ib) and recommendation (A). The use of short courses of oral steroids is indicated in patients with severe disease or in those patients with a mild to moderate disease who do not respond to topical steroids.

ACKNOWLEDGMENTS

The authors thank Danielle Creenaune (Australia) for the English revision of the manuscript.

REFERENCES

1. Benninger MS, Ferguson BJ, Hadley JA, et al. Adult chronic rhinosinusitis: definitions, diagnosis, epidemiology, and pathophysiology. Otolaryngol Head Neck Surg 2003;129(Suppl 3):S1–32.
2. Meltzer EO, Hamilos DL, Hadley JA, et al. Rhinosinusitis: establishing definitions for clinical research and patient care. J Allergy Clin Immunol 2004;114(suppl 6): S155–212.
3. Fokkens W, Lund V, Mullol J, et al. EP^{3}OS 2007: European position paper on rhinosinusitis and nasal polyps 2007. Rhinology 2007;20:1–136.
4. GINA 2006 Workshop Report: Global strategy for asthma management and prevention. WHO/NHLBI workshop report: National Institutes of Health, National Heart, Lung and Blood Institute, Publication Number 95-3659.
5. Bousquet J, van Cauwenberge P, Aït Khaled N, et al. Pharmacologic and anti-IgE treatment of allergic rhinitis. ARIA Update (in collaboration with GA^{2}LEN). Allergy 2006;61(9):1086–96.
6. Bousquet J, Khaltaev N, Cruz AA, et al. Allergic rhinitis and its impact on asthma (ARIA) 2008 update (in collaboration with the World Health Organization, GA2-LEN and AllerGen). Allergy 2008;63(suppl 86):8–160.
7. Pujols L, Mullol J, Torrego A, et al. Glucocorticoid receptors in human airways. Allergy 2004;59(10):1042–52.
8. Rhen T, Cidlowski JA. Antiinflammatory action of glucocorticoids—new mechanisms for old drugs. N Engl J Med 2005;353(16):1711–23.
9. Ray A, Siegel MD, Prefontine KE, et al. Anti-inflammation: direct physical association and functional antagonism between transcription factor NF-KB and the glucocorticoid receptor. Chest 1995;107(suppl 3):139S.
10. König H, Ponta H, Rahmsdorf HJ, et al. Interference between pathway-specific transcription factors: glucocorticoids antagonize phorbol ester-induced AP/1 activity without altering AP-1 site occupation in vivo. EMBO J 1992;11(6):2241–6.
11. Barnes PJ, Adcock IM. Glucocorticoid resistance in inflammatory diseases. Lancet 2009;373(9678):1905–17.
12. Pujols L, Mullol J, Roca-Ferrer J, et al. Expression of glucocorticoid receptor alpha- and beta-isoforms in human cells and tissues. Am J Physiol Cell Physiol 2002;283(4):C1324–31.
13. Pujols L, Mullol J, Picado C. Alpha and beta glucocorticoid receptors: relevance in airway diseases. Curr Allergy Asthma Rep 2007;7(2):93–9.
14. Pujols L, J Mullol, C Picado. Importance of glucocorticoid receptors in upper and lower airways. Front Biosci, in press.
15. Pujols L, Mullol J, Benitez P, et al. Expression of the glucocorticoid receptor alpha and beta isoforms in human nasal mucosa and polyp epithelial cells. Respir Med 2003;97(1):90–6.
16. Pujols L, Mullol J, Pérez M, et al. Expression of the human glucocorticoid receptor a and b isoforms in human respiratory epithelial cells and their regulation by dexamethasone. Am J Respir Cell Mol Biol 2001;24(1):49–57.
17. Pujols L, Alobid I, Benítez P, et al. Regulation of glucocorticoid receptor in nasal polyps by systemic and intranasal glucocorticoids. Allergy 2008; 63(10):1377–86.
18. Valotis A, Högge P. Human receptor kinetics and lung tissue retention of the enhanced-affinity glucocorticoid fluticasone furoate. Respir Res 2007;8(1):54.
19. Derendorf H, Meltzer EO. Molecular and clinical pharmacology of intranasal corticosteroids: clinical and therapeutic implications. Allergy 2008;63(10):1292–300.

20. Corren J. Intranasal corticosteroids for allergic rhinitis: how do different agents compare? J Allergy Clin Immunol 1999;104(4):S144–9.
21. Lipworth BJ, Seckl JR. Measures for detecting systemic bioactivity with inhaled and intranasal corticosteroids. Thorax 1997;52(5):476–82.
22. Szefler SJ. Pharmacokinetics of intranasal corticosteroids. J Allergy Clin Immunol 2001;108(Suppl 1):S26–31.
23. Lund VJ, Flood J, Sykes AP, et al. Effect of fluticasonein severe polyposis. Arch Otolaryngol Head Neck Surg 1998;124(5):513–8.
24. Vendelo Johansen L, Illum P, Kristensen S, et al. The effect of budesonide (Rhinocort) in the treatment of small and medium-sized nasal polyps. Clin Otolaryngol 1993;18(6):524–7.
25. Holmberg K, Juliusson S, Balder B, et al. Fluticasone propionate aqueous nasal spray in the treatment of nasal polyposis. Ann Allergy Asthma Immunol 1997; 78(3):270–6.
26. Small CB, Hernandez J, Reyes A, et al. Efficacy and safety of mometasone furoate nasal spray in nasal polyposis. J Allergy Clin Immunol 2005;116(6): 1275–81.
27. Benitez P, Alobid I, De Haro J, et al. A short course of oral prednisone followed by intranasal budesonide is an effective treatment of severe nasal polyps. Laryngoscope 2006;116(5):770–5.
28. Mygind N, Pedersen CB, Prytz S, et al. Treatment of nasal polyps with intranasal beclomethasone dipropionate aerosol. Clin Allergy 1975;5(2):159–64.
29. Deuschl H, Drettner B. Nasal polyps treated by beclomethasone nasal aerosol. Rhinology 1977;15(1):17–23.
30. Lildholdt T, Rundcrantz H, Lindqvist N. Efficacy of topical corticosteroid powder for nasal polyps: a double-blind, placebo-controlled study of budesonide. Clin Otolaryngol 1995;20(1):26–30.
31. Stjarne P, Blomgren K, Caye-Thomasen P, et al. The efficacy and safety of once-daily mometasone furoate nasal spray in nasal polyposis: a randomized, double-blind, placebo controlled study. Acta Otolaryngol 2006;126(6):606–12.
32. Alobid I, Benítez P, Bernal-Sprekelsen M, et al. Nasal polyposis and its impact on quality of life: comparison between the effects of medical and surgical treatments. Allergy 2005;60(4):452–8.
33. Aukema AA, Mulder PG, Fokkens WJ. Treatment of nasal polyposis and chronic rhinosinusitis with fluticasone propionate nasal drops reduces need for sinus surgery. J Allergy Clin Immunol 2005;115(5):1017–23.
34. Radenne F, Lamblin C, Vandezande LM, et al. Quality of life in nasal polyposis. J Allergy Clin Immunol 1999;104(1):79–84.
35. Rowe-Jones JM, Medcalf M, Durham SR, et al. Functional endoscopic sinus surgery: 5 year follow up and results of a prospective, randomised, stratified, double-blind, placebo controlled study of postoperative fluticasone propionate aqueous nasal spray. Rhinology 2005;43(1):2–10.
36. Dingsor G, Kramer J, Olsholt R, et al. Flunisolide nasal spray 0.025% in the prophylactic treatment of nasal polyposis after polypectomy. A randomized, double blind, parallel, placebo controlled study. Rhinology 1985;23(1):49–58.
37. Cuenant G, Stipon JP, Plante-Longchamp G, et al. Efficacy of endonasal neomycin-tixocortol pivalate irrigation in the treatment of chronic allergic and bacterial sinusitis. ORL J Otorhinolaryngol Relat Spec 1986;48(4):226–32.
38. Sykes DA, Wilson R, Chan KL, et al. Relative importance of antibiotic and improved clearance in topical treatment of chronic mucopurulent rhinosinusitis. A controlled study. Lancet 1986;2(8503):359–60.

39. Parikh A, Scadding GK, Darby Y, et al. Topical corticosteroids in chronic rhinosinusitis: a randomized, double-blind, placebo-controlled trial using fluticasone propionate aqueous nasal spray. Rhinology 2001;39(2):75–9.
40. Lavigne F, Cameron L, Renzi PM, et al. Intrasinus administration of topical budesonide to allergic patients with chronic rhinosinusitis following surgery. Laryngoscope 2002;112(5):858–64.
41. Lund VJ, Black JH, Szabó LZ, et al. Efficacy and tolerability of budesonide aqueous nasal spray in chronic rhinosinusitis patients. Rhinology 2004;42(2):57–62.
42. Cave A, Arlett P, Lee E. Inhaled and nasal corticosteroids: factors affecting the risks of systemic adverse effects. Pharmacol Ther 1999;83(3):153–79.
43. Holm AF, Fokkens WJ, Godthelp T, et al. A 1-year placebo-controlled study of intranasal fluticasone propionate aqueous nasal spray in patients with perennial allergic rhinitis: a safety and biopsy study. Clin Otolaryngol 1998;23(1):69–73.
44. Ernst P, Baltzan M, Deschênes J, et al. Low-dose inhaled and nasal corticosteroid use and the risk of cataracts. Eur Respir J 2006;27(6):1168–74.
45. Licata AA. Systemic effects of fluticasone nasal spray: report of 2 cases. Endocr Pract 2005;11(3):194–6.
46. Mehle ME. Are nasal steroids safe? Curr Opin Otolaryngol Head Neck Surg 2003; 11(3):201–5.
47. Schenkel EJ, Skoner DP, Bronsky EA, et al. Absence of growth retardation in children with perennial allergic rhinitis after one year of treatment with mometasone furoate aqueous nasal spray. Pediatrics 2000;105(2):E22.
48. Skoner D. Update of growth effects of inhaled and intranasal corticosteroids. Curr Opin Allergy Clin Immunol 2002;2(1):7–10.
49. Salib RJ, Howarth PH. Safety and tolerability profiles of intranasal antihistamines and intranasal corticosteroids in the treatment of allergic rhinitis. Drug Saf 2003; 26(12):863–93.
50. Van Camp C, Clement PA. Results of oral steroid treatment in nasal polyposis. Rhinology 1994;32(1):5–9.
51. Hissaria P, Smith W, Wormald PJ, et al. Short course of systemic corticosteroids in sinonasal polyposis: a double-blind, randomized, placebo-controlled trial with evaluation of outcome measures. J Allergy Clin Immunol 2006;118(1):128–33.
52. Walsh LJ, Lewis SA, Wong CA, et al. The impact of oral corticosteroid use on bone mineral density and vertebral fracture. Am J Respir Crit Care Med 2002; 166(5):691–5.
53. Becker SS, Rasamny JK, Han JK, et al. Steroid injection for sinonasal polyps: the University of Virginia experience. Am J Rhinol 2007;21(1):64–9.
54. McGrew RN, Wilson RS, Havener WH. Sudden blindness secondary to injections of common drugs in the head and neck: I. Clinical experiences. Otolaryngology 1978;86(1):147–51.
55. Scadding GK. Corticosteroids in the treatment of pediatric allergic rhinitis. J Allergy Clin Immunol 2001;108(suppl 1):S59–64.
56. Fokkens WJ, Scadding GK. Perennial rhinitis in the under 4s: a difficult problem to treat safely and effectively? A comparison of intranasal fluticasone propionate and ketotifen in the treatment of 2-4-year-old children with perennial rhinitis. Pediatr Allergy Immunol 2004;15(3):261–6.
57. Baena-Cagnani CE. Safety and tolerability of treatments for allergic rhinitis in children. Drug Saf 2004;27(12):883–98.
58. Al Sayyad JJ, Fedorowicz Z, Alhashimi D, et al. Topical nasal steroids for intermittent and persistent allergic rhinitis in children. Cochrane Database Syst Rev 2007;24(1):CD003163.

59. Pedersen S. Assessing the effect of intranasal steroids on growth. J Allergy Clin Immunol 2001;108(suppl 1):S40–4.
60. Skoner DP, Gentile D, Angelini B, et al. The effects of intranasal triamcinolone acetonide and intranasal fluticasone propionate on short-term bone growth and HPA axis in children with allergic rhinitis. Ann Allergy Asthma Immunol 2003; 90(1):56–62.
61. Agertoft L, Pedersen S. Short-term lower leg growth rate in children with rhinitis treated with intranasal mometasone furoate and budesonide. J Allergy Clin Immunol 1999;104(5):948–52.
62. Allen DB, Meltzer EO, Lemanske RF Jr, et al. No growth suppression in children treated with the maximum recommended dose of fluticasone propionate aqueous nasal spray for one year. Allergy Asthma Proc 2002;23(6):407–13.
63. Möller C, Ahlström H, Henricson KA, et al. Safety of nasal budesonide in the long-term treatment of children with perennial rhinitis. Clin Exp Allergy 2003;33(6): 816–22.
64. Skoner DP, Maspero J, Banerji D, et al. Assessment of the long-term safety of inhaled ciclesonide on growth in children with asthma. Pediatrics 2008;121(1): e1–14.
65. Skoner DP, Rachelefsky GS, Meltzer EO, et al. Detection of growth suppression in children during treatment with intranasal beclomethasone dipropionate. Pediatrics 2000;105(2):E23.
66. Kallen B, Rydhstroem H, Aberg A. Congenital malformations after the use of inhaled budesonide in early pregnancy. Obstet Gynecol 1999;93(3):392–5.
67. Schatz M, Zeiger RS, Harden K, et al. The safety of asthma and allergic medications during pregnancy. J Allergy Clin Immunol 1997;100(3):301–6.
68. Ellegard EK, Hellgren M, Karlsson NG. Fluticasone propionate aqueous nasal spray in pregnancy rhinitis. Clin Otolaryngol 2001;26(5):394–400.
69. Rodriguez-Pinilla E, Martinez–Frias ML. Corticosteroids during pregnancy and oral clefts. A case control study. Teratology 1998;58(1):2–5.
70. Einarson A, Bailey B, Jung S, et al. Prospective controlled study of hydroxyzine and cetirizine in pregnancy. Ann Allergy Asthma Immunol 1997;78(2):183–6.
71. Lehrer S, Sotne J, Lapinski R, et al. Association between pregnancy-induced hypertension and asthma during pregnancy. Am J Obstet Gynecol 1993; 168(5):1463–6.
72. Meltzer E, Hamilos D, Hadley J, et al. Rhinosinusitis: developing guidance for clinical trials. J Allergy Clin Immunol 2006;118(Suppl 5):S17–61.
73. Joe S, Thambi R, Huang J. A systematic review of the use of intranasal steroids in the treatment of chronic rhinosinusitis. Otolaryngol Head Neck Surg 2008;139(3): 340–7.

Aspirin Intolerance: Does Desensitization Alter the Course of the Disease?

L. Klimek, MD, PhD*, O. Pfaar, MD

KEYWORDS

- Samter triad • Morbus samter • Nasal polyps
- Aspirin sensitive • Aspirin intolerance
- Aspirin desensitization

In 1902, shortly after aspirin (acetylsalicylic acid [ASA]) was invented, cases of severe anaphylactoid reactions after aspirin ingestion were described by Hirschberg.[1] In 1922, Widal and colleagues[2] were the first to portray the association of aspirin sensitivity, aspirin-induced asthma (AIA), and nasal polyposis. The full clinical picture was subsequently pointed out in studies by Samter and Beers.[3] In many cases, nasal polyps reveal as the first symptom of ASA sensitivity.[4] This might indicate that the upper airways are predominantly involved in the pathogenetic process. Hence, the emphasis of this article is on the upper airways in ASA-intolerant patients.

ACETYLSALICYCLIC ACID INTOLERANCE: EICOSANOIDS AND THE ARACHIDONIC ACID METABOLISM

In the last decade, knowledge concerning the pathophysiologic mechanisms underlying ASA intolerance has been focused on in several studies. Evidence was found that the pathogenesis of aspirin intolerance is not an IgE-mediated reaction, but is related to an abnormal metabolism of arachidonic acid implicating both the lipoxygenase (LO) and the cyclooxygenase (COX) pathways.[4,5] This deviation results in a imbalance of the synthesis of eicosanoids, leukotrienes, and prostaglandins. Anti-inflammatory prostaglandins, especially E2, decrease; and the synthesis of cysteinyl-leukotrienes, such as leukotrien-A4, -B4, -C4 and -D4, is increased.[5,6]

PREVALENCE OF ACETYLSALICYCLIC ACID INTOLERANCE

Aspirin intolerance is thought to be underestimated. In a population of 500 patients with AIA studied in the European Network of Aspirin-Induced Asthma, 18% were

Center for Rhinology and Allergy, An den Quellen 10, D-65183 Wiesbaden, Germany
* Corresponding author.
E-mail address: ludger.klimek@allergiezentrum.de (L. Klimek).

Immunol Allergy Clin N Am 29 (2009) 669–675
doi:10.1016/j.iac.2009.07.008
0889-8561/09/$ – see front matter © 2009 Published by Elsevier Inc.

unaware of aspirin intolerance before having aspirin challenge tests.[7] More interesting, when patients with AIA also suffered from concomitant rhinosinusitis, 34% were unaware of their disease before testing.[8,9] Other data reveal incidence rates from 0.6% to 2.5% and, in adult asthmatics, from 4.3 % to 11%.[8]

CLINICAL SIGNS

In most cases, sensitivity to ASA reveals a typical pattern: rhinitis often becomes the first clinical sign during the third decade, often after a viral respiratory infection. After some months, concomitant chronic nasal congestion, hyposmia, chronic rhinorrhea, and nasal polyps might appear.[8,9] Finally, the disease results in AIA. Twenty percent of AIA patients suffer from mild and intermittent asthma, 30% are moderate asthmatics who can be controlled with inhaled steroids, and 50% of the patients have a chronic, severe corticoid-dependent asthma often accompanied by systemic anaphylactoid reactions.[9]

Upper-airways: The Key Area of Acetylsalicyclic Acid Intolerance

Rhinosinusitis was found to be a predominating symptom in 500 ASA-intolerant patients in a multicenter survey by Szczeklik and Nizankowska.[10] Nasal symptoms revealed at an average age of 30 years, often as a result of a viral respiratory infection. In these cases, the discharge of the nose was perennial and often watery. Hyposmic sensations were found in 55%. On average, the first asthmatic symptoms appeared two years later.

Nasal Polyps

In 70% of ASA-intolerant patients, nasal polyps can be found; whereas in the general population the overall prevalence of nasal polyps is only about 4%.[10,11] Typical for the polyps in ASA-intolerant patients is their aggressive growth that involves all paranasal sinuses bilaterally.[12] By means of CT-scans, Pansinus infection could be radiologically proven in almost all cases with AIA.[9]

The exact mechanisms of aspirin intolerance and those of therapy by ASA desensitization remain unclear. Evidence has been worked out that ASA intolerance is not an IgE-mediated reaction, but is related to an abnormal metabolism of arachidonic acid implicating both the LO and the CO pathways. This deviation results in a imbalance of the synthesis of the eicosanoids toward a predominance of the proinflammatory leukotrienes.[5,6]

The pathogenetic link between ASA intolerance and the origin of nasal polyps remains unclear. Infectious agents like viruses, bacteria, or fungi as potential primary factors might activate nasal epithelial cells and proinflammatory cytokines such as eotaxin and growth factors, thereby promoting the inflammatory process.[11,13,14] Other possible explanations might be differences in HLA genes,[15] a reduced apoptosis rate of local inflammation cells (eg, eosinophils[16]), or a differential role of COX-1 and COX-2 having special regulatory functions in the pathogenesis of nasal polyps.[17]

The recurrence rate of nasal polyps after resection in ASA-intolerant patients is tremendously high. In a study by Jantii-Alanco and colleagues,[18] the reoccurrence rate is almost three times higher in AIA than in non-intolerant intrinsic asthmatics.

DIAGNOSIS

Four typical findings in the patient''s history might correspond to intolerance to aspirin and other nonsteroidal antiinflammatory drugs (NSAIDs): (1) typical symptoms of respiratory reactions after aspirin challenge, (2) asthma attacks accompanied by chronic nasal congestion and watery, profuse rhinorrhea, (3) high frequency of severe asthmatic attacks, and (4) high frequency of nasal polyps.[5–7]

So far, validated and reliable in-vitro tests are not available for the diagnosis of aspirin intolerance. Provocation testing still is the only validated diagnostic tool for aspirin sensitivity. Nevertheless, challenge tests undoubtedly are harmful and should only be performed in specialized clinics well prepared for cases of anaphylactic reactions. Four types of aspirin challenge can be performed depending on the manner of administration: oral, inhalant, nasal, and intravenous.[7]

In cases of predominant nasal symptoms, a nasal challenge test with aspirin might be the method of choice because of its safety and its reliability.[19] In case of a negative test result in nasal challenge testing, but strong suspicions for AIA in the patient's history, bronchial or oral challenge tests should follow.[5,7]

THERAPY
Prevention of Selective COX-1

General rules concerning the treatment of AIA are related to the published guidelines on the management of asthma. Moreover, asthma attacks in AIA often result in a severe, potentially life-threatening course. This underlines the importance of educating the patients in avoiding ASA and all other cross-reacting, nonselective COX-inhibitors.[5,6] However, selective COX-2 inhibitors might be used safely in the majority of aspirin-sensitive patients.[20]

SURGERY

Massive growth of polyps in the nasal and paranasal-sinuses are resected by endoscopic or microscopic techniques. However, the recurrence rate is quite high. In a prospective study of 227 patients operated on for nasal polyposis between 1993 and 2001, a significantly higher rate of recurrences has been revealed in the AIA group compared with patients tolerant to ASA.[21]

ACETYLSALICYCLIC ACID DESENSITIZATION (ASPIRIN DESENSITIZATION, ADAPTIVE DESENSITIZATION)

In 1976, Zeiss and Lockey[22] described the paradoxical finding that ASA-intolerant patients revealed a 3-day refractory period after oral aspirin challenge. This report marked a new therapeutic option in the management of aspirin sensitive patients. Is it possible to treat the inflammatory airway-process with exactly the same medication which undoubtedly caused the symptoms? Based on these findings, various desensitization protocols and routes of administration have been elaborated on in the last 2 decades: bronchial, endonasal, oral, and (recently published) intravenous.

Bronchial Administration

This route of administration has been developed on the premise that refractory tolerance could be achieved by repeated provocation with lysine-aspirin inhalation.[23]

Endonasal Administration

In case of predominating nasal symptoms such as rhino-nasal polyposis, this route of administration has shown efficacy. In a study by Patriarca and colleagues,[24] intranasal desensitization was performed on 43 patients suffering from nasal polyposis with increasing doses of lysine acetylsalicylate corresponding to 20, 200, and 2000 micrograms of aspirin until a maximum dose of 2000 micrograms weekly was reached. In a 5-year follow up, recurrence rates of nasal polyps were significantly lower in the aspirin-treated group compared with the control group. Another randomized, double-blind, placebo-controlled, crossover trial of topical desensitization with a low-dose (16 mg) intranasal administration in 11 aspirin-sensitive, nasal polyp patients has been reported.[25] This study revealed only a poor clinical effect by the endonasal desensitization therapy. but significant improvement at the microscopic level.

Oral Administration

Stevenson and colleagues,[26] were the first to describe two cases of AIA patients who underwent an initial desensitization with incremental doses of aspirin followed by daily therapy. Interestingly, both patients revealed an improvement of the aspirin-sensitive asthma and a reduction of the nasal polyps. Only 4 years later, the same group published the first randomized, double-blind, placebo-controlled, crossover trial of aspirin desensitization in 25 patients with aspirin-sensitive asthma with a daily dosage between 325 and 1300 mg over a 3 month period.[27] This survey could demonstrate both a significant improvement of rhino nasal symptoms and a reduced need for nasal corticosteroids in the ASA-treated group compared with placebo. Nevertheless, only half of the patients experienced an improvement of their asthma symptoms.

One hundred and seven patients with diagnosed aspirin sensitivity with rhinosinusitis symptoms and AIA were involved in a retrospective survey published 6 years later.[28] In this study, 65 patients were treated by aspirin desensitization whereas a control group of 42 patients avoided all nonsteroidal antiinflammatory drugs (NSAIDs). Taken together, these data clearly demonstrate the clinical benefit of the desensitization therapy for aspirin-sensitive patients including a reduction in the number of hospitalizations and emergency room visits, upper-airway tract infections, and sinus operations; and an improvement in olfactory sense. Twenty percent of the 65 patients of the therapy group reported gastric complaints. Between 1988 and 1994, a long-term, follow-up study on aspirin desensitization with a daily peroral dose of 1300 mg was inaugurated.[29]

The importance of this study was the finding that aspirin desensitization reduces the aggressive growth and recurrence rate of sinunasal polyps in aspirin-sensitive patients over a longer period. The necessity for a sinunasal surgery declined from one operation every 3 years to one operation every 9 years. However, the number of emergency room visits and need for inhalable corticosteroids remained unchanged. A subsequent study with a similar design on 172 patients demonstrated a reduction of purulent sinusitis from an average of 5 times per year before therapy to les than half of

Table 1
Adaptive desensitization by IV application on patients with low-grade-intolerance

Day (Hospitalization)	Daily Dose of Lysine-Aspirin in mg (Given Bid, Morning and Afternoon)	
1	50	50
2	100	100
3	200	200
4	300	400
5	400	500
Maintenance-dose (outpatient)	300 mg aspirin daily, po	

Data from Pfaar O, Spielhaupter M, Wrede H, et al. Aspirin desensitization on patients with aspirin intolerance and nasal polyps. A new therapeutic approach by the intravenous route. Allergologie 2006;8:322–31.

Table 2		
Adaptive desensitization by IV application on patients with high-grade-intolerance		
Day (Hospitalization)	**Daily Dose of Lysine-Aspirin in mg (Given Bid, Morning and Afternoon)**	
1	25	25
2	50	50
3	100	100
4	200	200
5	300	400
6	400	500
Maintenance-dose (outpatient)	300 mg aspirin daily oral, po	

Data from Pfaar O, Spielhaupter M, Wrede H, et al. Aspirin desensitization on patients with aspirin intolerance and nasal polyps. A new therapeutic approach by the intravenous route. Allergologie 2006;8:322–31.

that.[30] A clinical response to treatment by 67% of patients was evident as early as 6 months, which indicates an early therapeutic effect of the desensitization therapy. Furthermore, these results persisted for 1 to 5 years. On the other hand, 9% discontinued the long-term therapy because of gastric symptoms, which was lower compared with the data of the same group from 1996.[29] The authors related these findings to the use of misoprostol and proton pump inhibitors, which became available in recent years.

Intravenous Administration

Recently, the intravenous (IV) route for ASA desensitization has been introduced into clinical practice.[31] N = 36 patients with a clear, positive history of ASA-intolerance, recurrent sinunasal polyps, and a positive test result in an oral challenge procedure and in an ex vivo test assay[32] were treated by ascending doses of intravenous lysine-aspirin under hospital conditions (**Tables 1** and **2**). The total amount of systemic reactions observed was n = 27 or 6.6% of all therapeutic doses. Of all systemic reactions, 81% were first-degree reactions and 19% second-degree reactions. Systemic reactions of the third or fourth degree have not been revealed.

Taken together, this survey indicated that the intravenous route for the initial ascending phase of ASA desensitization might be a safe procedure without severe complications comparable to the peroral route. In contrast to the peroral application, the intravenous procedure might have the advantage of interrupting the ASA application by stopping the infusion therapy in case of beginning systemic reactions. Undoubtedly, more studies are necessary to investigate the IV application concerning its safety aspects and comparability to the peroral application in the early phase of therapy.

SUMMARY

ASA desensitization is the only treatment that has shown to interfere with the natural course of ASA-intolerance syndrome (Samter's disease). Today, we have good evidence that desensitization reduces the growth and recurrence rate of nasal polyps in aspirin-sensitive patients over a longer period. The necessity for sinus surgery declined and the need for nasal corticosteroids had been reduced. The effect on symptoms, medication need. and exacerbation rate of bronchial asthma in ASA-intolerant patients is not as consistent as the effect on the upper airways. It was proposed

30 years ago that aspirin-precipitated reactions result from inhibition of COX by aspirin-like drugs in the airways or the skin of hypersensitive patients.[33] This basic COX theory has been restricted recently to COX-1 enzyme. Inhibition of COX-1 diminishes the synthesis of prostaglandin E2, normally acting as a brake on the production of cysteinyl leukotrienes (cysLTs).[4] Another distinguishing feature of aspirin hypersensitivity is the upregulation of the 5-lipoxygenase pathway, resulting in cysLT overproduction.[32,34]

In the beginning of ASA desensitization, a refractory status to aspirin or NSAIDs was thought to be the mechanism of action of this therapeutic approach. Now, however, there is more and more evidence for regulatory effects of ASA desensitization.

Based on recent clinical and laboratory data, the authors hypothesize that ASA desensitization leads to a quantitative or qualitative induction of cyclooxygenases, especially COX-1. These enzymes are quantitatively reduced or inactive in ASA-intolerant patients even without the intake of aspirin or other NSAIDs. Therefore, ASA desensitization does alter the natural course of the disease.

REFERENCES

1. Hirschberg VG. Anaphylactoid reaction to aspirin (1902). (classical article). Allergy Proc 1990;11:249–52.
2. Widal MF, Abrami P, Lenmoyez J. Anaphylaxie et idiosyncrasie. Presse Med 1922; 30:189–92.
3. Samter M, Beers RF. Intolerance to aspirin. Clinical studies and consideration of its pathogenesis. Ann Intern Med 1968;68:975–83.
4. Szczeklik A, Stevenson DD. Aspirin-induced asthma: advances in pathogenesis, diagnosis, and management. J Allergy Clin Immunol 2003;111:913–21.
5. Babu KS, Salvi S. Aspirin and asthma. Chest 2000;118:1470–8.
6. Pfaar O, Klimek L. Aspirin desensitization in aspirin intolerance: update on current standards and recent improvements. Curr Opin Allergy Clin Immunol 2006;6:161–6.
7. Szczeklik A, Nizankowska E, Duplaga M. Natural history of aspirin-induced asthma. AIANE Investigators. European Network on Aspirin-Induced Asthma. Eur Respir J 2000;16(3):432–6.
8. Szczeklik A, Sanak M, Niz E, et al. Aspirin intolerance and the cyclooxygenase-leukotriene pathways. Curr Opin Pulm Med 2004;10:51–6.
9. Berges-Gimeno MP, Simon RA, Stevenson DD. The natural history and clinical characteristics of aspirin-exacerbated respiratory disease. Ann Allergy Asthma Immunol 2002;89(5):474–8.
10. Szczeklik A, Nizankowska E. Clinical features and diagnosis of aspirin-induced asthma. Thorax 2000;55(Suppl 2):42–4.
11. Bachert C, Watelet JB, Gevaert P, et al. Pharmacological management of nasal polyposis. Drugs 2005;65(11):1537–52.
12. Picado C, Mullol J. The nose in aspirin-sensitive asthma. In: Szczeklik A, Gryglewski RJ, Vane J, editors. Eicosanois, aspirin and asthma. New York: Marcel Dekker; 1998. p. 493–505.
13. Pawliczak R, Lewandowska-Polak A, Kowalski ML. Pathogenesis of nasal polyps: an update. Curr Allergy Asthma Rep 2005;6:463–71.
14. Min JW, Jang AS, Park SM, et al. Comparison of plasma eotaxin family level in aspirin-induced and aspirin-tolerant asthma patients. Chest 2005;128(5): 3127–32.
15. Molnar-Gabor E, Endreffy E, Rozsasi A. HLA-DRB1, -DQA1, and -DQB1 genotypes in patients with nasal polyposis. Laryngoscope 2000;110(3 Pt 1):422–5.

16. Kowalski ML, Grzegorczyk J, Pawliczak R, et al. Decreased apoptosis and distinct profile of infiltrating cells in the nasal polyps of patients with aspirin hypersensitivity. Allergy 2002;57(6):493–500.

17. Gosepath J, Brieger J, Mann WJ. New immunohistologic findings on the differential role of cyclooxygenase 1 and cyclooxygenase 2 in nasal polyposis. Am J Rhinol 2005;19(2):111–6.

18. Jantii-Alanco S, Holopainen E, Malmberg H. Recurrence of nasal polyps after surgical treatment. Rhinology 1989;8:59–64.

19. Milewski M, Mastalerz L, Nizankowska E. Nasal provocation test with lysine-aspirin for diagnosis of aspirin-sensitive asthma. J Allergy Clin Immunol 1998; 101:581–6.

20. Stevenson DD, Simon RA. Lack of cross-reactivity between rofecoxib and aspirin-sensitive patients with asthma. J Allergy Clin Immunol 2001;108:47–51.

21. Albu S, Tomescu E, Mexca Z, et al. Recurrence rates in endonasal surgery for polyposis. Acta Otorhinolaryngol Belg 2004;58(1):79–86.

22. Zeiss CR, Lockey RF. Refractory period to aspirin in a patient with aspirin-induced asthma. J Allergy Clin Immunol 1976;57(5):440–8.

23. Schmitz-Schumann M, Schaub E, Virchow C. Inhalation provocation test with lysineacetylsalicylic acid in patients with analgetics-induced asthma. Prax Klin Pneumol 1982;36(1):17–21.

24. Patriarca G, Schiavino D, Nucera E, et al. Prevention of relapse in nasal polyposis. Lancet 1991;337(8755):1488.

25. Parikh AA, Scadding GK. Intranasal lysine-aspirin in aspirin-sensitive nasal polyposis: a controlled trial. Laryngoscope 2005;115(8):1385–90.

26. Stevenson DD, Simon RA, Mathison DA. Aspirin-sensitive asthma: tolerance to aspirin after positive oral aspirin challenges. J Allergy Clin Immunol 1980;66: 82–8.

27. Stevenson DD, Pleskow WW, Simon RA, et al. Aspirin-sensitive rhinosinusitis asthma: a double blind cross over study of treatment with aspirin. J Allergy Clin Immunol 1984;73:500–7.

28. Sweet J, Stevenson DD, Simon RA, et al. Long-term effects of aspirin desensitization—treatment for aspirin-sensitive rhinosinusitis-asthma. J Allergy Clin Immunol 1990;85:59–65.

29. Stevenson DD, Hankammer MA, Mathison DA, et al. Aspirin desensitization treatment of aspirin-sensitive patients with rhinosinusitis-asthma: long-term outcomes. J Allergy Clin Immunol 1996;98(4):751–8.

30. Berges-Gimeno P, Simon RA, Stevenson DD. Long-term treatment with aspirin desensitization in asthmatic patients with aspirin-exacerbated respiratory disease. J Allergy Clin Immunol 2003;111:180–6.

31. Pfaar O, Spielhaupter M, Wrede H, et al. Aspirin desensitization on patients with aspirin intolerance and nasal polyps. a new therapeutic approach by the intravenous route. Allergologie 2006;8:322–31.

32. Schaefer D, Lindenthal U, Wagner M, et al. Effect of prostaglandin E2 on eicosanoid release by human bronchial biopsy specimens from normal and inflamed mucosa. Thorax 1996;51(9):919–23.

33. Szczeklik A, Gryglewski R, Czerniawska-Mysik G. Relationship of inhibition of prostaglandin biosynthesis by analgesics to asthma attacks in aspirin-sensitive patients. Br Med J 1975;1:67–9.

34. Christie P, Tagari P, Ford-Hutchinson AW, et al. Urinary leukotriene E4 concentrations increase after aspirin challenge in aspirin-sensitive asthmatic subjects. Am Rev Respir Dis 1991;143:1025–9.

Fungus: A Role in Pathophysiology of Chronic Rhinosinusitis, Disease Modifier, A Treatment Target, or No Role at All?

Wytske J. Fokkens, MD, PhD*, Fenna Ebbens, MD, PhD,
Cornelis M. van Drunen, PhD

KEYWORDS

- Rhinosinusitis • Paranasal sinus diseases • Physiopathology
- Diagnosis • Therapy • Fungus

According to the position paper on chronic rhinosinusitis (CRS) by EP[3]OS 2007,[1] CRS (including nasal polyps) is defined as: an inflammation of the nose and the paranasal sinuses characterized by 2 or more symptoms, one of which should be either nasal blockage/obstruction/congestion or nasal discharge (anterior/posterior nasal drip) combined with facial pain/pressure, and/or reduction or loss of smell; and either endoscopic signs of polyps, and/or mucopurulent discharge primarily from middle meatus, and/or edema/mucosal obstruction primarily in middle meatus, and/or computed tomography (CT) changes like mucosal changes within the ostiomeatal complex and/or sinuses.[1] CRS is considered to be a multifactorial disease in which a large number of factors may eventually lead to impaired ciliary function, more mucus with increased viscosity, and mucosal swelling, resulting in symptoms of CRS. CRS is also considered to be a common denominator for several diseases that cannot or only with great difficulty be differentiated clinically.

Patients with CRS with and without nasal polyps can be differentiated clinically, although even this differentiation is not always easy. Also, sometimes with help of the pathologist or laboratory measurements one is able to discriminate some causes of CRS as exists in different forms of vasculitis, Wegener disease, or cystic fibrosis.

Department of Otorhinolaryngology, Academic Medical Center (AMC), Meibergdreef 9, 1100 AZ Amsterdam, The Netherlands
* Corresponding author.
E-mail address: w.j.fokkens@amc.nl (W. J. Fokkens).

Immunol Allergy Clin N Am 29 (2009) 677–688
doi:10.1016/j.iac.2009.07.002

After removal of all identifiable causes of CRS, a large group of clinically indistinguishable patients remain, in which it is presumed that one or more factors contribute to the disease.

MICROORGANISMS

Microorganisms have always been popular suspects in the pathophysiology of CRS. Almost all microorganisms have been mentioned: in some patients the microorganism is a likely cause of the disease, for example, in fulminant fungal disease in patients with immunodeficiencies. In other situations, such as involving *Staphylococcus aureus*, an aggravating or disease-modifying factor seems to be a more plausible explanation.

This article focuses on the potential role of fungi in CRS. In which situations are fungi a plausible cause? Can fungi be a disease modifier or do they not play a role at all?

FUNGUS

Fungal spores, due to their ubiquitous nature, are continuously inhaled and deposited on the airway mucosa. Although they rarely behave as pathogens in the airways of healthy individuals, they may cause human disease in some. Five forms of fungal disease affecting the nose and paranasal sinuses have been recognized to date: (1) acute invasive fungal rhinosinusitis (including rhinocerebral mucormycosis), (2) chronic invasive fungal rhinosinusitis, (3) granulomatous invasive fungal rhinosinusitis, (4) fungal ball (mycetoma), and (5) noninvasive (allergic) fungal rhinosinusitis[2] (adapted from DeShazo and Swain[3]). Invasive forms of fungal rhinosinusitus are considered to be rare and generally occur in immunocompromised hosts only. Noninvasive forms of fungal rhinosinusitis, rare but slightly more common than invasive forms, include sinus mycetoma (fungal ball), in general affecting only one sinus, and noninvasive (allergic) fungal rhinosinusitis, affecting multiple sinuses. The latter 2 generally occur in immunocompetent individuals.

FUNGUS IN IMMUNOCOMPETENT INDIVIDUALS

In this article the authors focus on the role of fungi in immunocompetent individuals, as most patients do not seem to have an obvious immunodeficiency. Fungal spores, due to their ubiquitous nature, are continuously inhaled and deposited on the airway mucosa. In this review the authors try to follow the fungus from mucus to epithelium with innate and acquired nasal immune responses, and the potential secondary response to the fungus, to determine what potential role it might play in the pathogenesis of CRS.

Like the paranasal sinuses, the entire nasal cavity is lined by a thin layer of respiratory mucosa composed of ciliated, pseudostratified, columnar epithelial cells with goblet mucous cells interspersed among the columnar cells. A deep layer of mucus covers the entire nasal cavity. This mucus is slightly acidic and consists of 2 layers: a thin, low-viscosity, periciliary layer (sol phase) that envelops the cilia of the columnar cells, and a thick, more viscous layer (gel phase) riding on the periciliary layer. The distal tips of the ciliary shafts contact the gel layer and move particulate matter, inhaled bacteria, and fungi that are caught in this gel layer toward the nasopharynx. The presence of fungi due to a disturbance in the process of inhalation, retention, and clearance of fungal spores begins as soon as the spores make contact with the airway, and must be differentiated from fungal-related diseases of the paranasal sinuses.

Novel culture techniques, first described by Ponikau and colleagues, resulted first in a prevalence rate of almost 100% in mucus of CRS patients[4] and not much later in most of the normal controls as well.[5,6] What was learned from these studies is that fungal spores are everywhere and that if the detection method is sensitive enough, fungi can be found in every patient and control. Now most investigators agree that the polymerase chain reaction is superior to both culture and Grocott methanamine silver stains in detecting fungal elements.[7]

Thus fungal elements are a normal phenomenon in the nasal mucus but, despite this constant exposure to fungi, fungal disease of the nasal sinuses is relatively rare. Even if one would argue that all cases of CRS are caused by fungi, not more than around 10% of the population would be affected. A high degree of coexistence normally would seem to occur between fungi and their mammalian hosts, which deviates into overt disease under conditions of too low or too high immune responses.[8] The ubiquitous presence of fungi in the nose and paranasal sinuses of both CRS patients and healthy controls could lead to the argument that it is not the presence or absence of fungi, but rather a specific fungal species or fungal load that is relevant for disease development. Cultures collected via the novel technique described previously[4] grew 37 to 40 different genera with 2.7 to 3.2 species per CRS patient and 2.3 to 3.1 per healthy control.[4–6] *Aspergillus*, *Penicillium*, *Cladosporium*, *Candida*, *Aureobasidium*, and *Alternaria* appeared most frequently, with no significant differences between the 2 groups. A different study, assessing the amount of fungal DNA present in tissue specimens obtained from CRS patients and healthy controls, demonstrated no differences in fungal load between the 2 groups,[9] rendering it unlikely that fungal species and fungal load play a role in disease development. Whether an increase in fungal allergen content is involved in CRS pathogenesis remains unclear.

Just as in allergens, fungi may contain proteolytic activity, which may diminish epithelial integrity and thus expose the epithelium to fungal elements. Thus mechanical barriers, effective mucociliary clearance, and optimal healing limit the degree of antigenic stimulation of immune cells residing in the mucosa. Despite this impressive barrier function, animate and inanimate matter will stimulate the mucosal immune system, which must distinguish between commensal organisms and potential invading pathogens without excessive tissue damage. Two distinct but integrated immune responses to microbial entities and foreign proteins have been described: innate and acquired. This article focuses first on the innate immunity.

COULD DYSFUNCTIONAL MUCUS BE A REASON FOR FUNGAL DISEASE IN THE NASAL SINUS?

The major macromolecular constituents of mucus are the mucin glycoproteins. Mucins are secreted by mucous epithelial goblet and glandular cells, and themselves contribute important antimicrobial and anti-inflammatory properties.

Furthermore, multiple substances with antimicrobial and immunomodulatory actions, such as surfactant proteins and antimicrobial peptides, are secreted by the epithelial cells, local inflammatory cells, and submucosal glands, resulting in killing of the fungus. Recent proteomics research has shown interesting differences in the expression of proteins related to regulation of immune cells and mediators in mucus of CRS patients compared with controls.[10,11] Data on the function of these proteins are still limited but some interesting data, mainly from the group of Wormald, have recently appeared.

Various antimicrobial peptides have been shown to play a role in fungal elimination and have been identified in mucus of CRS patients. This group of peptides consists among others of lactoferrin, lysozyme and secretory leukoprotease inhibitor, surfactant proteins, and cathelicidins and defensins.[12]

Lactoferrin possesses a variety of functions, including antimicrobial and antibiofilm properties.[13,14] Bacterial biofilms are present in most CRS patients, and may contain large amounts of fungal elements.[15] Downregulation of lactoferrin was recently observed in those CRS patients with nasal polyps[16] or those with biofilms.[17] However, no difference was observed between CRS patients with or without eosinophilic mucin, those with or without fungal allergy, and those with or without fungi present.[16,17]

Cathelicidins and defensins are 2 major families of cationic antimicrobial peptides involved in innate immunity at mucosal surfaces. Ooi and colleagues[18] recently demonstrated that LL-37, the free C-terminal peptide of human cathelicidin hCAP18 (human cationic antimicrobial peptide 18 kDa), is significantly upregulated in a dose-response effect at the mRNA and protein level in CRS patients without eosinophilic mucin in response to Aspergillus fumigatus and Alternaria tenuis. However, in CRS patients with eosinophilic mucin (but without fungal presence), no significant increase in LL-37 was observed at either the mRNA or the protein level in response to Aspergillus challenge. No increase in expression in both tissue and secreted LL-37 was observed on Alternaria challenge. Although the idea is interesting, because neither CRS patients with eosinophilic mucin and fungal presence nor a control group were included in this study, the exact role of LL-37 in the CRS pathogenesis remains to be determined.

Pulmonary surfactant is a mixture of phospholipids and proteins. Four different surfactant proteins (SPs) are known to exist: SP-A, SP-B, SP-C, and SP-D.[19] SP-D binds and agglutinates microorganisms and enhances phagocytosis, chemotaxis, and cytokine production. SP-D has been shown to play an important role in the immune response to Aspergillus fumigatus in the lung and is present in submucosal glands of CRS patients without eosinophilic mucin, CRS patients with eosinophilic mucin but without fungal allergy and healthy controls. Highest levels are detected in healthy controls. In CRS patients with eosinophilic mucin and fungal allergy, SP-D protein levels are below the detection level. In vitro studies demonstrate that Alternaria tenuis upregulates SP-D mRNA in those CRS patients with and those without eosinophilic mucin. Aspergillus fumigatus, on the other hand, increases SP-D mRNA expression in CRS patients without eosinophilic mucin only.[20] Absence of SP-D protein may result in failure to clear fungi from the nose and paranasal sinuses and, as a result, disease development. In conclusion, the mucus and proteins secreted in the mucus are an important part of the innate immunity. The first data on dysfunction of this system are yet to appear. For the moment, cause and effect relationships are unclear.

WHAT HAPPENS WHEN THE FUNGUS REACHES THE EPITHELIUM?

The epithelial layer occupies a strategic important location between an organism's interior and exterior environment. Although as such it forms a physical barrier between both environments, it has become clear that the role of the epithelium extends far beyond this passive role. Through specialized receptors and other more general mechanisms, the epithelial layer is not only able to sense changes in its environment but also to actively respond to these changes.

The receptors of the innate immunity on the epithelial cells have only a limited specificity, and can be activated by interaction with common protein motives or pathogen-associated molecular patterns found in microorganisms like fungi. The Toll-like receptors (TLR) are probably the best studied group of pattern recognition receptors. In most vertebrates, the Toll family comprises about 10 family members with a highly conserved intracellular signaling domain that resembles the signaling domain found in the mammalian interleukin (IL)-1 receptor. All TLRs activate a core set of stereotyped responses, such as inflammation. However, individual TLRs can also induce specific programs in cells of the innate immune system that are tailored for the particular pathogen. For the innate immunity reaction to fungi, TLR2, 4, and 6 seem to be the most important.[21] There are limited data on the expression pattern of the TLRs in the upper airway and even less functional data. Variable expression for TLR2 and TLR4 was found in tissue samples from patients with CRS with and without nasal polyposis compared with controls, but most studies indicate a lower expression, which might result in a reduced ability of the epithelium to react to and eliminate fungal antigen.[22–26]

Epithelial cells from CRS patients have also been shown to have poor TLR2-induced release of neutrophil-attracting chemokines such as IL-8.[26,27] It is unclear as to the exact role of TLRs and whether they contribute to a reduced or a changed reaction to fungi in CRS patients.

Fungi have important protease activity. In this way they can activate epithelial cells via their protease-activated receptors (PARs). Activation of nasal epithelial cells with fungi results in an upregulation of PAR2 and PAR3 mRNAs.[28] Proteases present in fungal extracts like *Alternaria* have been shown to interact with epithelial cells, most likely through a PAR2 receptor driven mechanism leading to morphologic changes, cell desquamation, and induction of proinflammatory cytokines like IL-6 and IL-8.[29] These proinflammatory cytokines are then able to attract and stimulate neutrophils, and stimulate further inflammation. However, through this mechanism eosinophilic inflammation does not seem to be induced; in at least one study in CRS patients PAR2 stimulation did not lead to release of eosinophil attracting cytokines like eotaxin or RANTES.[30] IL-6 is a key cytokine, mediating the transition from innate to acquired immunity, possibly acting by dampening the innate response, and fostering the acquired response. One key component of IL-6 action is that this cytokine frees helper and effector T cells from the suppressive effects of IL-10 secreted by Treg.[27] The local increase in IL-6, by PAR2 stimulation, might result in an inhibition of local innate immune responses and may also dampen local adaptive immunosuppression mediated through Treg cells.[27]

PAR receptors are not only found on epithelial cells but also on inflammatory cells like neutrophils and eosinophils, which leads to the question of cellular response to fungi in CRS.

CELLULAR IMMUNE RESPONSE TO FUNGI IN CHRONIC RHINOSINUSITIS

Cellular immune responses vary according to the fungal species, the morphotype encountered, and the anatomic site of interaction. Whereas yeasts and spores are often effectively phagocytosed, the larger size of hyphae precludes effective ingestion and requires interaction with different inflammatory cells. Neutrophils, macrophages, and monocytes are important antifungal effector cells. However, in CRS almost all attention focuses on the role of eosinophils.

Fungi and Eosinophils

Eosinophils are an important hallmark of CRS, especially with nasal polyps, in the Western world.[31,32] The concurrent presence of fungi and eosinophils in nearly all CRS tissue specimens has led to the suggestion of a cause and effect relationship.[33,34] In follow-up studies a concentration-dependent increase in (CRS) eosinophil migration toward both CRS nasal mucin and CRS nasal tissue extracts was shown,[35] and peripheral blood mononuclear cells (PBMCs) from CRS patients exposed to *Alternaria* fungal extracts generated a mixed Th1/Th2 cytokine profile, whereas cells from normal patients did not respond.[36] Also, a component of *Alternaria* was shown to degranulate eosinophils from CRS patients by acting on PARs, suggesting that fungi may trigger inflammatory cells to initiate a complex localized eosinophilic reaction.[37] These data were interpreted to be consistent with a T-cell–driven, non-IgE–mediated response that resulted in the attraction and specific targeting of eosinophils against colonized fungi in the nasal lumen of CRS patients, with subsequent degranulation and mucosal damage implying an acquired immune response. However, several challenges can be made to this hypothesis. First, probably most important, no specific T-cell receptor responses to fungal antigens that are unique in CRS have been shown to date, raising the question whether the induced reactions were the results of nonspecific protease effects of the *Alternaria* extract on PBMCs already activated by the concurrent allergy or asthma rather than fungal antigen presentation and T-cell responses.[36] Of note, 14 out of 18 patients in this study were asthmatic compared with none of the controls. Fungal extracts have established nonspecific protease effects,[21] and it is totally unclear whether the used concentration of extract was in the same range as could be expected in vivo.

Moreover, activated eosinophils from subjects with asthma (both allergic and nonallergic asthma) are known to exhibit by themselves a primed phenotype that is likely the consequence of eosinophil interaction with cytokines in the peripheral blood, resulting in increased eosinophil migration-, adhesion-, and degranulation capacities, so also for this reason it may well be that the presence of asthma or atopy rather than that of fungi explains the observed concentration-dependent increase in eosinophil migration.[38,39] This hypothesis is supported by recent data in sheep, in which primed eosinophils were shown to be more effective in immobilizing and killing gastrointestinal parasites in the presence of specific antiparasite antibodies in comparison with unprimed eosinophils,[40] and also because a second study (in which the frequency of atopy was equally distributed) showed only minimal changes in IL-5 and interferon-γ expression on culture with *Aspergillus* and *Alternaria* extracts.[41]

T Cells and Fungus

CRS has been subdivided by some investigators into a neutrophilic/Th1 disease without nasal polyps and an eosinophilic/Th2 disease with nasal polyps. However, recent data showing a discrepancy in nasal polyp formation and eosinophilia in Asian polyps and European polyps in patients with cystic fibrosis challenge this hypothesis. Cystic fibrosis nasal polyps and non-Caucasian nasal polyps, polyps macroscopically remarkably similar to Caucasian nasal polyps, are characterized by abundant tissue neutrophilia and not tissue eosinophilia.[42–44]

Recent findings in experimental candidiasis and aspergillosis shed new light on the contribution of Th17 cells to resistance and pathology to fungi. It has been shown that resistance and tolerance to fungi are 2 types of host defense mechanisms to increase fitness in response to fungi.[45] In experimental candidiasis and aspergillosis, both defense mechanisms are activated through the delicate equilibrium between Th1 cells (which provide antifungal resistance mechanisms) and Treg, limiting the consequences of the associated inflammatory pathology.[8] In the studies determining a possible role for fungus in CRS, no difference is recognized between CRS with and without nasal polyps. However, different types of inflammation (Th1, Th2, and Treg) could result in disturbed T17 regulation. Data on IL-17 in CRS are not consistent. Increased IL-17-positive cells, and increased expression of IL-17 and its receptor have been reported in Caucasian CRS without nasal polyps (CRSwNP),[46,47] although these data could not be confirmed by others.[27,48] It has been shown recently by the same group that contrary to CRSwNP from Caucasian patients, nasal polyps from Asian patients demonstrated a T(h)1/T(h)17 polarization. A protective role of Th17 cells and IL-17A in defense against fungal infection has been implicated.[49] However, Zelante and colleagues suggest that IL-23 and IL-17A have a largely negative role in fungal infection. Gene deletion or neutralization of IL-23 and IL-17A improved immunopathology and fungal control after pulmonary *Aspergillus fumigatus* infection. Stimulation of neutrophils with IL-23 or IL-17A led to impaired fungicidal activity along with increased secretion of matrix metalloproteinase (MMP)-9 and myeloperoxidase.[8] Both these mediators are found to be increased in chronic rhinosinusitis.[44,50] Zelante and colleagues point to a detrimental effect in the course of fungal infections at the mucosal surfaces of Th17 responses by affecting fungal clearance, and by promoting chronic inflammation and tissue damage.[8] The relationship between chronic inflammation, T-cell regulation, and the potential role of fungi is far from clear; as has been stated before, specific T-cell responses to fungi in CRS have not been shown to date, but a detrimental effect of fungi on the inflamed sinus mucosa via T-cell regulation cannot be excluded.

Is There a Role for Fungal-Specific IgG?

If acquired immunity to fungi plays a role in CRS, one might expect humoral defense mechanisms to be activated. Increased levels of fungal-specific IgG and IgA, specifically IgG1 and IgG3 isotypes to fungi in CRS patients with eosinophilic mucin, have been described irrespective of the presence of specific IgE antibodies in the nasal polyp tissue or the concomitant serum.[51,52] These findings suggest that increases in fungal antigen-specific antibodies of different isotypes reflect the individual's ability to mount a nonallergic humoral immune response. However, the way in which the fungal-specific IgG might contribute to the inflammation is unclear. A direct role in the activation or degranulation of eosinophils does not seem very likely.[51] For now, other than being a biologic marker for CRS patients with eosinophilic mucin, the pathogenic significance of fungal-specific IgG remains undetermined.

Is Type I Hypersensitivity to Fungi Involved in the Pathogenesis of Chronic Rhinosinusitis?

Various investigators have studied sensitization rates to fungi in CRS patients and controls, demonstrating values ranging from 18% to 46%, and usually no difference between CRS patients and healthy controls[4] or patients with allergic rhinitis.[52] Also, the presence of fungal antigen-specific IgE does not seem to distinguish noninvasive fungal rhinosinusitis patients from other CRS patients, and there are no data indicating that allergy to certain fungi species are specifically relevant.[36,52,53]

However, similar to allergic bronchopulmonary aspergillosis, an allergic reaction to fungi also in the upper airways has been proposed as a cause of disease: allergic fungal rhinosinusitis (AFS). Based on the finding that only three-fourths of patients diagnosed with AFS were atopic, the role of type 1 hypersensitivity[3] and later also the need for a positive fungal histology has been disputed. Therefore one should bear in mind that the criteria used to define AFS differs between various studies, although most investigators agree on a positive fungal histology or culture, eosinophilic mucin, and CT findings consistent with CRS. Considering this line of thought, is was not strange that Ponikau and colleagues, based on the fact that fungi can be cultured from every patient (and control), proposed that fungi might be the cause of all forms of CRS. In all patients with CRS 2 of the 3 prerequisites for AFS seem to be fulfilled. All patients do have abnormalities on CT scan, and culturing fungi is possible in the mucus of all patients with CRS (as in all healthy controls). The only thing left is the eosinophilic mucus. What exactly is eosinophilic mucus? Eosinophilic mucus has been described to have a distinct macroscopic appearance, being thick, tenacious, and dark colored.[54] Eosinophils are the predominant and a consistent cellular component that defines eosinophilic mucus; eosinophil breakdown products

(Charcot-Leyden crystals), sloughed respiratory epithelial cells, and debris are also present.[54] So thick, dark-colored mucus with eosinophils were the first hallmarks of the disease; fungal elements were not always found.[55,56] The International Society for Human and Animal Mycology recently convened a working group to attempt consensus on terminology and disease classification. The working group has concluded that allergic fungal rhinosinusitis (AFRS), eosinophilic fungal rhinosinusitis, and eosinophilic mucin rhinosinusitis (EMRS) are imprecise and require better definition, and propose that to implicate fungi (as in AFRS and EMRS), hyphae must be visualized in eosinophilic mucin, but they also indicate that this is often not processed or examined carefully enough by histologists, reducing the universality of the disease classification.[57] Also, whether the combination of eosinophils and hyphae point to an allergic reaction to the fungi is questionable. So although the assumption of a unique pathogenic role of fungal allergy in noninvasive fungal rhinosinusitis should be questioned, there might be a role for concurrent fungal allergy in some CRS patients.

Does Reduction of Fungal Load Improve Symptoms in Chronic Rhinosinusitis?

Despite initial evidence of benefit in 2 uncontrolled trials,[58,59] one subsequent uncontrolled prospective trial[60] and 4 subsequent double-blind placebo-controlled studies investigating the effect of topical amphotericin B nasal lavage[61–63] and nasal sprays[60,64] in CRS patients with and without nasal polyposis either failed to show benefit[60,61,63,64] or showed, at best, only modest nonrelevant radiological benefit without symptomatic improvement.[62]

Although all randomized controlled trials until now do not support the use of topical antifungals in the treatment of CRS with or without nasal polyposis, dosage, treatment time, and route of administration may have influenced treatment outcomes. As recent in vitro data suggest that amphotericin B nasal lavages are ineffective in killing fungi at concentrations of 100 μg/mL when used for 6 consecutive weekly dosages used by both Ponikau and colleagues[58] and the authors' group,[61,65] a lack of effect may be explained by inadequate dosing. Although inadequate dosing of topical amphotericin B may explain the observed results, treatment with topical amphotericin B at a concentration of 250 μg/mL, a dose that was demonstrated to be effective in killing fungi, was shown to be ineffective as well.[62]

What Mechanisms of Antifungal Treatment Exist to Reduce Symptoms in Chronic Rhinosinusitis?

Although reduction of fungal load seems to be the most obvious potential mechanism to explain fungal treatment, Weschta and colleagues showed that fungal eradication does not alleviate CRS signs and symptoms.[64] However, amphotericin B may also have a direct (cytotoxic) effect on nasal polyp epithelial cells. Although amphotericin B is a sterol-binding agent with high affinity for ergosterol (the dominant fungal sterol) and low affinity for cholesterol (the mammalian sterol), recent evidence suggests that topical amphotericin B, though at dosages higher than used in most clinical studies, is able to modify cell membrane structures of nasal polyp epithelial cells, resulting in increased membrane permeability and disruption of cells.[66] A third potential mechanism could be a direct anti-inflammatory effect of amphotericin B on the CRS mucosa. Although interesting, to date no studies exist confirming this hypothesis. At the moment no data support one of the potential mechanisms described earlier. Studies published to date report no difference between placebo- and amphotericin B-treated patients at the concentrations of various proinflammatory cytokines, chemokines, and growth factors.[65,67,68]

SUMMARY

There are several potential deficits in the innate and potentially also acquired immunity of CRS patients that might reduce or change their ability to react to fungi. There are not many arguments to suggest a causative role for fungi in CRS with or without nasal polyps. However, due to the intrinsic or induced change in immunity of CRS patients, fungi might have a disease-modifying role. The inability to reduce symptoms and signs of CRS inflammation by antifungal treatment, however, moderates one's enthusiasm to put a lot of effort into further unraveling this role.

REFERENCES

1. Fokkens W, Lund V, Mullol J. EP[3]OS 2007: European position paper on rhinosinusitis and nasal polyps 2007. A summary for otorhinolaryngologists. Rhinology 2007;45(2):97–101.
2. Ebbens FA, Georgalas C, Rinia AB, et al. The fungal debate: where do we stand today? Rhinology 2007;45(3):178–89.
3. deShazo RD, Swain RE. Diagnostic criteria for allergic fungal sinusitis. J Allergy Clin Immunol 1995;96(1):24–35.
4. Ponikau JU, Sherris DA, Kern EB, et al. The diagnosis and incidence of allergic fungal sinusitis. Mayo Clin Proc 1999;74(9):877–84.
5. Kim ST, Choi JH, Jeon HG, et al. Comparison between polymerase chain reaction and fungal culture for the detection of fungi in patients with chronic sinusitis and normal controls. Acta Otolaryngol 2005;125(1):72–5.
6. Murr AH, Goldberg AN, Vesper S. Fungal speciation using quantitative polymerase chain reaction (QPCR) in patients with and without chronic rhinosinusitis. Laryngoscope 2006;116(8):1342–8.
7. Ebbens FA, Georgalas C, Fokkens WJ. The mold conundrum in chronic hyperplastic sinusitis. Curr Allergy Asthma Rep 2009;9(2):114–20.
8. Zelante T, De Luca A, D'Angelo C, et al. IL-17/Th17 in anti-fungal immunity: what's new? Eur J Immunol 2009;39(3):645–8.
9. Scheuller MC, Murr AH, Goldberg AN, et al. Quantitative analysis of fungal DNA in chronic rhinosinusitis. Laryngoscope 2004;114(3):467–71.
10. Tewfik MA, Latterich M, DiFalco MR, et al. Proteomics of nasal mucus in chronic rhinosinusitis. Am J Rhinol 2007;21(6):680–5.
11. Casado B, Pannell LK, Iadarola P, et al. Identification of human nasal mucous proteins using proteomics. Proteomics 2005;5(11):2949–59.
12. Ooi EH, Wormald PJ, Tan LW. Innate immunity in the paranasal sinuses: a review of nasal host defenses. Am J Rhinol 2008;22(1):13–9.
13. Cavestro GM, Ingegnoli AV, Aragona G, et al. Lactoferrin: mechanism of action, clinical significance and therapeutic relevance. Acta Biomed 2002;73(5–6):71–3.
14. Singh PK, Parsek MR, Greenberg EP, et al. A component of innate immunity prevents bacterial biofilm development. Nature 2002;417(6888):552–5.
15. Healy DY, Leid JG, Sanderson AR, et al. Biofilms with fungi in chronic rhinosinusitis. Otolaryngol Head Neck Surg 2008;138(5):641–7.
16. Psaltis AJ, Bruhn MA, Ooi EH, et al. Nasal mucosa expression of lactoferrin in patients with chronic rhinosinusitis. Laryngoscope 2007;117(11):2030–5.
17. Psaltis AJ, Wormald PJ, Ha KR, et al. Reduced levels of lactoferrin in biofilm-associated chronic rhinosinusitis. Laryngoscope 2008;118(5):895–901.
18. Ooi EH, Wormald PJ, Carney AS, et al. Fungal allergens induce cathelicidin LL-37 expression in chronic rhinosinusitis patients in a nasal explant model. Am J Rhinol 2007;21(3):367–72.

19. Crouch E, Hartshorn K, Ofek I. Collectins and pulmonary innate immunity. Immunol Rev 2000;173:52–65.

20. Ooi EH, Wormald PJ, Carney AS, et al. Surfactant protein d expression in chronic rhinosinusitis patients and immune responses in vitro to *Aspergillus* and *Alternaria* in a nasal explant model. Laryngoscope 2007;117(1):51–7.

21. Vroling AB, Fokkens WJ, van Drunen CM. How epithelial cells detect danger: aiding the immune response. Allergy 2008;63(9):1110–23.

22. Dong Z, Yang Z, Wang C. Expression of TLR2 and TLR4 messenger RNA in the epithelial cells of the nasal airway. Am J Rhinol 2005;19(3):236–9.

23. Claeys S, de Belder T, Holtappels G, et al. Human beta-defensins and toll-like receptors in the upper airway. Allergy 2003;58(8):748–53.

24. Pitzurra L, Bellocchio S, Nocentini A, et al. Antifungal immune reactivity in nasal polyposis. Infect Immun 2004;72(12):7275–81.

25. Lane AP, Truong-Tran QA, Schleimer RP. Altered expression of genes associated with innate immunity and inflammation in recalcitrant rhinosinusitis with polyps. Am J Rhinol 2006;20(2):138–44.

26. Wang J, Matsukura S, Watanabe S, et al. Involvement of Toll-like receptors in the immune response of nasal polyp epithelial cells. Clin Immunol 2007;124(3):345–52.

27. Kern RC, Conley DB, Walsh W, et al. Perspectives on the etiology of chronic rhinosinusitis: an immune barrier hypothesis. Am J Rhinol 2008;22(6):549–59.

28. Shin SH, Lee YH, Jeon CH. Protease-dependent activation of nasal polyp epithelial cells by airborne fungi leads to migration of eosinophils and neutrophils. Acta Otolaryngol 2006;126(12):1286–94.

29. Kauffman HF, Tomee JF, van de Riet MA, et al. Protease-dependent activation of epithelial cells by fungal allergens leads to morphologic changes and cytokine production. J Allergy Clin Immunol 2000;105(6 Pt 1):1185–93.

30. Rudack C, Steinhoff M, Mooren F, et al. PAR-2 activation regulates IL-8 and GRO-alpha synthesis by NF-kappaB, but not RANTES, IL-6, eotaxin or TARC expression in nasal epithelium. Clin Exp Allergy 2007;37(7):1009–22.

31. Bachert C, Van Bruaene N, Toskala E, et al. Important research questions in allergy and related diseases: 3-chronic rhinosinusitis and nasal polyposis—a GA-LEN study. Allergy 2009;64(4):520–33.

32. Zhang N, Holtappels G, Claeys C, et al. Pattern of inflammation and impact of *Staphylococcus aureus* enterotoxins in nasal polyps from southern China. Am J Rhinol 2006;20(4):445–50.

33. Ponikau JU, Sherris DA, Kephart GM, et al. Striking deposition of toxic eosinophil major basic protein in mucus: implications for chronic rhinosinusitis. J Allergy Clin Immunol 2005;116(2):362–9.

34. Ponikau JU, Sherris DA, Kephart GM, et al. Features of airway remodeling and eosinophilic inflammation in chronic rhinosinusitis: is the histopathology similar to asthma? J Allergy Clin Immunol 2003;112(5):877–82.

35. Wei JL, Kita H, Sherris DA, et al. The chemotactic behavior of eosinophils in patients with chronic rhinosinusitis. Laryngoscope 2003;113(2):303–6.

36. Shin SH, Ponikau JU, Sherris DA, et al. Chronic rhinosinusitis: an enhanced immune response to ubiquitous airborne fungi. J Allergy Clin Immunol 2004; 114(6):1369–75.

37. Inoue Y, Matsuwaki Y, Shin SH, et al. Nonpathogenic, environmental fungi induce activation and degranulation of human eosinophils. J Immunol 2005;175(8): 5439–47.

38. Griffin E, Hakansson L, Formgren H, et al. Increased chemokinetic and chemotactic responses of eosinophils in asthmatic patients. Allergy 1991; 46(4):255–65.

39. Koenderman L, van der Bruggen T, Schweizer RC, et al. Eosinophil priming by cytokines: from cellular signal to in vivo modulation. Eur Respir J Suppl 1996; 22:119s–25s.

40. Rainbird MA, Macmillan D, Meeusen EN. Eosinophil-mediated killing of *Haemonchus contortus* larvae: effect of eosinophil activation and role of antibody, complement and interleukin-5. Parasite Immunol 1998;20(2):93–103.

41. Douglas R, Bruhn M, Tan LW, et al. Response of peripheral blood lymphocytes to fungal extracts and staphylococcal superantigen B in chronic rhinosinusitis. Laryngoscope 2007;117(3):411–4.

42. Sobol SE, Christodoulopoulos P, Manoukian JJ, et al. Cytokine profile of chronic sinusitis in patients with cystic fibrosis. Arch Otolaryngol Head Neck Surg 2002; 128(11):1295–8.

43. Van Zele T, Claeys S, Gevaert P, et al. Differentiation of chronic sinus diseases by measurement of inflammatory mediators. Allergy 2006;61(11):1280–9.

44. Zhang N, Van Zele T, Perez-Novo C, et al. Different types of T-effector cells orchestrate mucosal inflammation in chronic sinus disease. J Allergy Clin Immunol 2008;122(5):961–8.

45. Romani L. Cell mediated immunity to fungi: a reassessment. Med Mycol 2008; 46(6):515–29.

46. Wang X, Dong Z, Zhu DD, et al. Expression profile of immune-associated genes in nasal polyps. Ann Otol Rhinol Laryngol 2006;115(6):450–6.

47. Molet SM, Hamid QA, Hamilos DL. IL-11 and IL-17 expression in nasal polyps: relationship to collagen deposition and suppression by intranasal fluticasone propionate. Laryngoscope Oct 2003;113(10):1803–12.

48. Van Bruaene N, Perez-Novo CA, Basinski TM, et al. T-cell regulation in chronic paranasal sinus disease. J Allergy Clin Immunol 2008;121(6):1435–41, 1441, e1431–3.

49. Acosta-Rodriguez EV, Rivino L, Geginat J, et al. Surface phenotype and antigenic specificity of human interleukin 17-producing T helper memory cells. Nat Immunol 2007;8(6):639–46.

50. Watelet JB, Bachert C, Claeys C, et al. Matrix metalloproteinases MMP-7, MMP-9 and their tissue inhibitor TIMP-1: expression in chronic sinusitis vs nasal polyposis. Allergy 2004;59(1):54–60.

51. Sabirov A, Hamilton RG, Jacobs JB, et al. Role of local immunoglobulin E specific for *Alternaria alternata* in the pathogenesis of nasal polyposis. Laryngoscope 2008;118(1):4–9.

52. Pant H, Kette FE, Smith WB, et al. Fungal-specific humoral response in eosinophilic mucus chronic rhinosinusitis. Laryngoscope 2005;115(4):601–6.

53. Collins MM, Nair SB, Wormald PJ. Prevalence of noninvasive fungal sinusitis in South Australia. Am J Rhinol 2003;17(3):127–32.

54. Katzenstein AL, Sale SR, Greenberger PA. Allergic *Aspergillus* sinusitis: a newly recognized form of sinusitis. J Allergy Clin Immunol 1983;72(1):89–93.

55. Lara JF, Gomez JD. Allergic mucin with and without fungus: a comparative clinicopathologic analysis. Arch Pathol Lab Med 2001;125(11):1442–7.

56. Ramadan HH, Quraishi HA. Allergic mucin sinusitis without fungus. Am J Rhinol 1997;11(2):145–7.

57. Chakrabarti A, Denning DW, Ferguson BJ, et al. Fungal rhinosinusitis: a categorization and definitional schema addressing current controversies. Laryngoscope 2009; in press.

58. Ponikau JU, Sherris DA, Kita H, et al. Intranasal antifungal treatment in 51 patients with chronic rhinosinusitis. J Allergy Clin Immunol 2002;110(6):862–6.

59. Ricchetti A, Landis BN, Maffioli A, et al. Effect of anti-fungal nasal lavage with amphotericin B on nasal polyposis. J Laryngol Otol 2002;116(4):261–3.

60. Helbling A, Baumann A, Hanni C, et al. Amphotericin B nasal spray has no effect on nasal polyps. J Laryngol Otol 2006;120(12):1023–5.

61. Ebbens FA, Scadding GK, Badia L, et al. Amphotericin B nasal lavages: not a solution for patients with chronic rhinosinusitis. J Allergy Clin Immunol 2006; 118(5):1149–56.

62. Ponikau JU, Sherris DA, Weaver A, et al. Treatment of chronic rhinosinusitis with intranasal amphotericin B: a randomized, placebo-controlled, double-blind pilot trial. J Allergy Clin Immunol 2005;115(1):125–31.

63. Liang KL, Su MC, Shiao JY, et al. Amphotericin B irrigation for the treatment of chronic rhinosinusitis without nasal polyps: a randomized, placebo-controlled, double-blind study. Am J Rhinol 2008;22(1):52–8.

64. Weschta M, Rimek D, Formanek M, et al. Topical antifungal treatment of chronic rhinosinusitis with nasal polyps: a randomized, double-blind clinical trial. J Allergy Clin Immunol 2004;113(6):1122–8.

65. Ebbens FA, Georgalas C, Luiten S, et al. The effect of topical amphotericin B on inflammatory markers in patients with chronic rhinosinusitis: a multicenter randomized controlled study. Laryngoscope 2009;119(2):401–8.

66. Jornot L, Rochat T, Lacroix JS. Nasal polyps and middle turbinates epithelial cells sensitivity to amphotericin B. Rhinology 2003;41(4):201–5.

67. Shin SH, Ye MK. Effects of topical amphotericin B on expression of cytokines in nasal polyps. Acta Otolaryngol 2004;124(10):1174–7.

68. Weschta M, Rimek D, Formanek M, et al. Effect of nasal antifungal therapy on nasal cell activation markers in chronic rhinosinusitis. Arch Otolaryngol Head Neck Surg 2006;132(7):743–7.

Anti-Inflammatory Effects of Macrolides: Applications in Chronic Rhinosinusitis

Richard J. Harvey, MD[a],*, Ben D. Wallwork, MD, PhD[b],
Valerie J. Lund, MD[c]

KEYWORDS

- Chronic • Sinusitis • Rhinosinusitis • Macrolides
- Immunomodulation • Interleukin • Neutrophilic

The anti-inflammatory effects of macrolides are significant. The clinical impact on diffuse panbronchiolitis (DPB) has improved 10-year survival from 12% to more than 90% for these patients.[1] Diffuse panbronchiolitis (DPB) was first reported in 1969 as a new chronic lung disease characterized by chronic recurrent bronchiolitis and peribronchiolitis, with infiltration of lymphocytes and plasma cells.[2] Obstruction of the small airways through the formation of lymphoid follicles, granulomas, and scars was part of the disease progression. Clinical features of DPB are productive cough, shortness of breath, and radiography with bilateral diffuse granular shadows. In addition, the titers of cold hemagglutinin are elevated to more than 64 times the normal value in these patients.[2] A predisposition to human leukocyte antigen (HLA) B54 is common in patients with DPB (63.2%), whereas it is present only in 11.4% of the normal healthy Japanese population.[3]

Since the first report of long-term macrolide therapy by Kudoh and colleagues in 1987,[4] similar efficacy has been reproduced for DPB.[1,5–7] With such a dramatic impact on DPB, the immunomodulatory impact of macrolides has been a source of mechanistic research as well as clinical research in non-DPB related inflammatory airway disease. The inflammatory mechanisms of chronic rhinosinusitis (CRS) have been a major non-DPB focus. Macrolides have been trialed in more than 14 prospective trials and are the focus of numerous research projects.[8] This article discusses the current concepts of the proposed activity of macrolides and their application in the management of CRS.

a Department of Otolaryngology, Skull Base Surgery, St. Vincent's Hospital, Sydney, NSW 2010, Australia
b Department of Otolaryngology, Princess Alexandra Hospital, Brisbane, QLD 4000, Australia
c Rhinology Research Unit, The Royal National Throat, Nose and Ear Hospital, Gray's Inn Road, London WC1X 8DA, United Kingdom
* Corresponding author.
E-mail address: richard@richardharvey.com.au (R. Harvey).

Immunol Allergy Clin N Am 29 (2009) 689–703
doi:10.1016/j.iac.2009.07.006   immunology.theclinics.com

MACROLIDES AS AN ANTIMICROBIAL

Macrolides are the natural or semisynthetic derivatives of the polyketides. Polyketides are natural secondary metabolites from bacteria, fungi, plants, and animals biosynthesized in a similar process to fatty acid synthesis.[9] The macrolide group of drugs gain their activity from the presence of a macrolide ring, a large macrocyclic lactone ring to which one or more deoxy sugars are attached (**Fig. 1**). The lactone rings are usually 14-, 15-, or 16-membered (**Fig. 2**). The macrolides predominantly include antibiotics, but also immunosuppressants such as the drugs tacrolimus and sirolimus, with a similar activity to cyclosporin.

Primary antibiotic activity involves the inhibition of bacterial protein biosynthesis by reversibly binding to the 50S subunit of bacterial ribosome. This binding inhibits the translation of peptidyl tRNA. The action is mainly bacteriostatic, but can also be bactericidal in high concentrations. Macrolides tend to accumulate within leukocytes, and are therefore actively transported into the site of infection.[10]

A broad range of bacteria are susceptible to macrolide antibiotics. Penicillins are considered the treatment of choice for group A β-hemolytic streptococcal infections of the upper respiratory tract, for example, acute rhinosinusitis, tonsillitis, or pharyngitis. A macrolide, mainly erythromycin, is indicated for the treatment of penicillin allergic patients. A therapeutic dose is usually administered for 10 days. In addition to *Streptococcus pyogenes and Streptococcus pneumoniae,* macrolides also have activity against *Haemophilus influenzae* (some strains are resistant) and *Staphylococcus aureus.* Other bacteria such as *Legionella pneumophila, Treponema pallidum, Neisseria gonorrhoeae, Listeria monocytogenes, Bordetella pertussis, Corynebacterium diphtheriae* (as an adjunct to antitoxin), *Campylobacter jejuni* (in severe or prolonged cases), and *Chlamydia trachomatis* are also susceptible.

BACTERIAL RESISTANCE

The primary means of bacterial resistance to macrolides occurs by posttranscriptional methylation of the 23S bacterial ribosomal RNA. Acquired resistance can be either plasmid-mediated or chromosomal, that is, through mutation, and results in cross-resistance to macrolides, lincosamides, and streptogramins. Two other uncommon types of acquired resistance include the production of drug-inactivating enzymes (esterases or kinases) and the production of active ATP-dependent efflux proteins that transport the drug outside of the cell.[11] A new class of antibiotics that are structurally related to the macrolides are the ketolides. Ketolides are used to fight respiratory tract infections caused by macrolide-resistant bacteria. Examples include telithromycin (Ketek), cethromycin, spiramycin (used for treating toxoplasmosis), ansamycin, oleandomycin, carbomycin, and tylocine. Large epidemiologic studies on the resistance patterns for telithromycin suggest that resistance has been

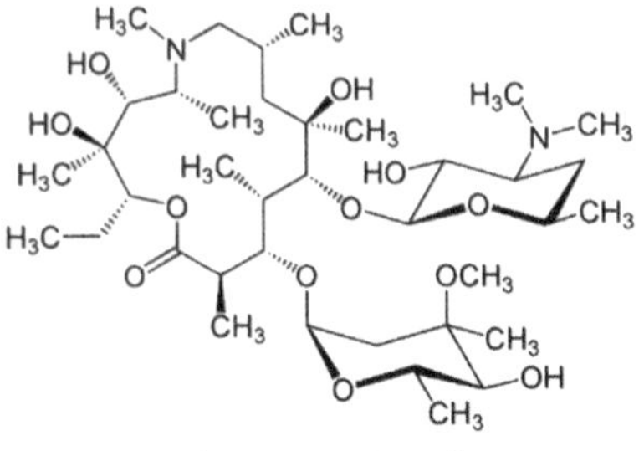

Fig. 1. The structure of azithromycin, demonstrating the macrocyclic lactone ring.

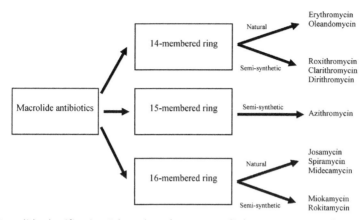

Fig. 2. Macrolide classification is based on the macrocyclic lactone ring, membered by deoxy sugars.

controllable.[12] The reported rate of high-level resistance was 5.7%[12] and comparable to the 3.4% reported in 1995.[13] Long-term use of macrolides in Japan for diffuse panbronchiolitis similarly has not been associated with the development of significant resistance.[5]

IMMUNOMODULATION VERSUS IMMUNOSUPPRESSION

Respiratory epithelial damage, mucus hypersecretion, mucociliary dysfunction, and the release of proinflammatory products at the sinus mucosa all mediate the prolonged inflammation of CRS.[14] The role of local microbial flora in CRS has shifted from one of causation to disease modifier.[15] Although there has been a shift to anti-inflammatory therapies in CRS,[16,17] bacteria and fungi are likely to be powerful mediators of inflammation, and an appropriate immune response may be beneficial even in the setting of CRS. 'The authors' current model of CRS pathophysiology focuses on the interaction of the inflammatory mucosal disease with bacteria, and the failure of the mechanical and innate immunity (**Fig. 3**).

The immune response in some conditions, such as multiple sclerosis, has long been simply linked to pathology but recent evidence suggests a neuroprotective role from the immune reaction.[18] Immunomodulatory therapies that target those responses which facilitate axonal loss may be more appropriate than blanket immunosuppression. In CRS, similarly, although antimicrobial therapy alone is not a therapy for CRS, blunt immunosuppression of the underlying neutrophilic or eosinophilic inflammation is unlikely to provide a simple solution. The human immune system has evolved as a complex nonlinear feedback system with extensive redundancy.[19] Classic immunosuppression from current medications, such as corticosteroids, may suppress components of the innate and mechanical immunity. Suppression of the entire system may not be the most appropriate way to achieve mucosal homeostasis. Immunomodulation rather than immunosuppression is the feature of the non-antimicrobial activity of macrolides and provides one therapeutic approach to the disordered inflammatory response in CRS.

BIOLOGIC EFFECTS

A significant body of research, in vivo and in vitro, has occurred over the past decade to better understand the immunomodulatory mechanisms induced by macrolides. The

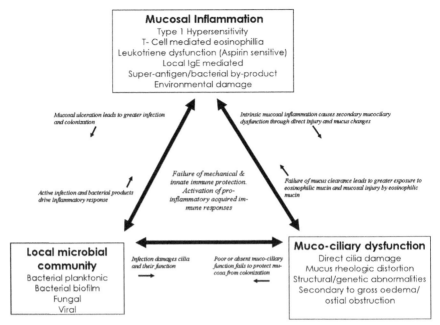

Fig. 3. The pathophysiologic interaction of intrinsic mucosal inflammation, microbial flora, and mucociliary dysfunction. Macrolides have effects across all 3 interacting processes: the ability to modulate the neutrophilic immune response, direct activity on bacteria, antibiofilm properties, and changes to mucus rheology and production. (*Courtesy of* Division of Rhinology, St. Vincent's Hospital; with permission.)

ability of macrolides to block the production of proinflammatory cytokines, such as interleukin (IL)-8 and tumor necrosis factor-α (TNF-α), combined with effects on neutrophil migration and adhesion, form the basis of their action. Additional immunomodulatory activity, changes to mucus secretion and synthesis, and nonbacteriostatic/-cidal microbial activity are also well described. It is likely that only the 14- and 15-membered ring macrolides have these additional properties.[20] Macrolides have the ability to modify all 3 contributing factors in the pathophysiology of CRS (see **Fig. 3**). Current non-antimicrobial characteristics of macrolides are summarized as immunomodulatory, mucin, and bacterial effects in the next sections (**Tables 1 and 2**).

Immunomodulatory

Macrolide pharmacokinetics produce an intracellular uptake and concentration. This concentration can be up to 100 times the serum level and occurs in neutrophils, macrophages, and fibroblasts.[21] This accumulation is also greater under cytokine stimulation and at inflammatory sites.[22]

Neutrophils

Modulation of neutrophilic action by macrolides is the most widely recognized in the bronchial and sinus mucosa.[23–27] Macrolides can suppress lipopolysaccharide (LPS) induced neutrophil migration and infiltration into mucosa in animal models.[28] This suppression was observed only in macrolide pretreatment and not amoxicillin. Neutrophil adhesion and the upregulation of intracellular adhesion molecule (ICAM) expression in response to LPS are thought to mediate part of this process. Macrolides

Table 1
Mechanisms of action of macrolide antibiotics in chronic respiratory disease

Target	Macrolide Action	In Vivo/In Vitro	First Author of Study, Year
Transcription factors	Suppression of NF-κB and AP-1	In vitro	Wallwork, 2002 Kikuchi, 2002
Cytokine production	Decreased IL-5, IL-8, GM-CSF Decreased TGF-β Decreased IL-6, IL-8, TNF-α	In vitro In vitro In vivo	Wallwork, 2004 Wallwork, 2002 Suzuki, 1997 Gao, 2007 Cigana, 2007
Cytokine production	Increased concentration of anti-inflammatory cytokines IL-1ra, IL-6, IL-10	In vivo	Tamaoki, 2004
Matrix metalloproteins	Reduction of matrix metalloproteinase-7	In vitro	Yasuda, 2007
Biofilm formation	Altered structure and function of biofilm	In vitro	Wozniak, 2004
Leukocyte adhesion	Reduced expression of cell surface adhesion molecules	In vitro	Linn, 2000
Apoptosis	Accelerate neutrophil apoptosis	In vitro	Inamura, 2000 Aoshiba, 1995
Oxidative burst	Impaired neutrophil oxidative burst	In vivo	Hand, 1990
Mucociliary clearance	Decreased secretions Improved clearance	In vitro	Rubin, 1997 Nishi, 1995
Bacterial Virulence	Inhibited release of elastase, protease, phospholipase C, and eotaxin A by *Pseudomonas aeruginosa*	In vitro	Hirakata, 1992
Viral entry into cell	Inhibit viral entry (protease inhibitor)	In vitro	Kido, 2007

Full references are available in the source article.
Abbreviations: AP, activator protein; GM-CSF, granulocyte macrophage-colony stimulating factor; IL, interleukin; NF-κB, nuclear factor-κB; TGF, transforming growth factor; TNF, tumor necrosis factor.
Data from Cervin A, Wallwork B. Anti-inflammatory effects of macrolide antibiotics in the treatment of chronic rhinosinusitis. Otolaryngol Clin North Am 2005;38:1339–50.

Table 2
The antibiofilm effects of macrolide therapy

Author	Macrolide	Main Findings
Hoffman et al, 2007[78]	Sub-MIC AZM	Block QS and alginate polymer formation, increase biofilm sensitivity in stationary growth phase
Nalca et al, 2006[54]	Sub-MIC AZM	Inhibition of QS activities, decrease motility and virulence factors in P aeruginosa
Woznidk and Keyser, 2004[53]	Sub-MIC CLA	↓ Twitching motility, change the structure of biofilm formation
Gillis and Iglewski, 2004[79]	Sub-MIC AZM	Delayed biofilm formation of P aeruginosa
Imanura et al, 2004[80]	AZM, CLA	Inhibits MUC5AC production induced by P aeruginosa via an inhibitory effect on the ERK pathway
Carter et al, 2004[81]	Sub-MIC CLA	Inhibit Mycobacterium avium biofilm formation if employed early, but no effects on established biofilm
Favre-Bonte et al, 2003[82]	AZM	↓ The production of both AHLs in the P aeruginosa biofilms
Tateda et al, 2001[83]	AZM (2 μg/mL)	Inhibition of QS
Kawamura-sato et al, 2000[84]	Sub-MIC of EM, CLA, AZM	↓ The expression of flagellin, inhibition of motility in P mirabilis and P aeruginosa
Mitsuya et al, 2000[56]	EM and MDM	↓ Biofilm formation by inhibiting GMD production cycle
Tateda et al, 2000[85]	Sub-MIC EM and AZM	↓ Protein synthesis, suppression of virulence factors, and stress response in P aeruginosa
Ichimiya et al, 1996[86]	AZM	↓ Alginate production
Mizukane et al, 1994[87]	AZM, EM, RXM, RKM	↓ Production of exotoxin A, total protease, elastase phospholipase
Yasuda et al, 1994[88]	Sub-MICs CLA	Eradication of slimelike structure, decrease in the quantity of hexose in S epidermidis
Yasuda et al, 1993	CLA (10 μg/mL)	Eradicate the membranous structures produced by P aeruginosa

Abbreviations: AHL, acyl homoserine lactone; AZM, azithromycin; CAM, clarithromycin; EM, erythromycin; GMD, guanosine diphospho-D-mannose dehydrogenase; QS, quorum sensing; RXM, roxithromycin; Sub-MIC, subminimal inhibitory concentration.

can suppress LPS-induced ICAM expression in a dose-dependent manner.[20] Additional downregulation of selectins, integrins, and other adhesion molecules are also reported.[29–31]

Macrolides reduce free radical production by neutrophils, and this occurs at drug levels that are unlikely to have an antimicrobial effect.[32] Whereas erythromycin may enhance superoxide dismutase activity,[33] azithromycin seems to clear superoxide by a mechanism unrelated to currently understood scavenging pathways.[34]

Interleukin-8

IL-8 is both a target for and product of neutrophils. IL-8 is a potent proinflammatory cytokine with neutrophil chemoattractant properties, and is released in response to LPS, TNF-α, and aggregated immune complexes.[20] IL-8 is thought to be a significant mediator of the inflammatory response in certain subtypes of CRS.[35] Fourteen- and 15-membered ring macrolides have been shown to impair the production of IL-8 in both lung and nasal tissue.[36,37] Macrolides are thought to reduce production of IL-8 by suppressing transcription factors. Nuclear factor (NF)-κB and activator protein (AP)-1 are transcription factors important in the inflammatory response, and inhibition of these factors can decrease the expression of IL-8 and other cytokines.[27] Erythromycin and clarithromycin have been shown to suppress IL-8 production by this process.[38,39] NF-κB and AP-1 are downregulated in response to clarithromycin[40] and erythromycin.[41] Intracellular cell signaling via the extracellular signal-regulated kinase (ERK) and p38 mitogen-activated protein kinase (MAPK) pathways are thought to mediate these transcription factors.[42]

Other cytokine production, mainly IL-5, transforming growth factor-β (TGF-β), and granulocyte macrophage-colony stimulating factor (GM-CSF), are also suppressed from clarithromycin use.[43,44] Th2 cytokine (IL-4 and IL-5) suppression and the effects on eosinophils have been demonstrated.[45,46] However, the effects on eosinophilic inflammation and in vivo responses are less convincing.[47]

Nitric Oxide

Nitric oxide (NO) is an important player in several normal physiologic airway processes but can also act as an inflammatory mediator. Neutrophils, respiratory epithelium, and macrophages have NO synthase and are capable of inducible NO production. Macrolide therapy can suppress the NO release from pulmonary macrophages after immune complex injury in rats.[48] Similar effects with cefaclor and amoxicillin were not observed.

Leukotrienes

Erythromycin has been shown to modulate the lipoxygenase pathway of arachidonic acid.[49] Leukotriene B4 (LTB4) is a powerful chemoattractant for neutrophils in DPB and other inflammatory airway diseases. Corresponding lower LTB4 and neutrophils are present in those patients on erythromycin therapy.[49]

BACTERIAL (NONRIBOSOMAL 50S RELATED) ACTIONS

The success of macrolide therapy in managing some patients with cystic fibrosis (CF) has spawned much research into alternative effects on bacteria. Gram-negative bacteria such as *Pseudomonas* are not readily susceptible to the 50s ribosomal bacteriostatic effects of macrolides. However, many of the virulence factors are affected by macrolides. Pseudomonal protease, elastase, phospholipase C, and eotaxin A are suppressed by erythromycin therapy.[50] Pseudomonal adherence to respiratory, buccal mucosa and type-4 collagen are all suppressed with erythromycin or azithromycin therapy.[51,52] Macrolides are believed to reduce biofilm formations through reduced twitching motility,[53] surface signaling,[54,55] and exopolysaccharide formation.[56] Quorum sensing and the initial phases of biofilm formation are thought to be affected by these mechanisms.[57] Clarithromycin has been shown to decrease viable bacteria within a biofilm despite not having a direct antibacterial effect.[58] A summary of macrolide activity on bacterial biofilms is presented in **Table 2**.

MUCUS
Mucus Secretion

There is a strong association with IL-8 mediated mucus release in animal models.[59] Roxithromycin and erythromycin have been shown to suppress this release, possibly through IL-8 mechanisms. Macrolides can reduce goblet cell secretion in response to LPS in animal models.[28] clarithromycin clinically decreased sputum expectoration by 50% in patients with DPB, chronic bronchitis, or bronchiectasis.[60] In CRS, macrolides have improved mucus clearance and production, and have reduced saccharine clearance time.[61,62] This effect is likely to result from alterations in mucus rheologic properties, thus creating more effective clearance.[62] High chloride content within some mucus samples may contribute to unfavorable rheologic properties, and macrolides have been shown in vivo[63] and in vitro[64] to reduce chloride content. This reduction may create more "watery" secretions.

Mucus Synthesis

High-density mucin glycoproteins define much of the elasticity and viscosity of airway mucus.[65] MUC4, MUC5AC, and MUC5B are major components of airway mucus. Macrolides inhibit MUC5AC mRNA in response to LPS by a similar mechanism to IL-8 suppression.[20] Similar effects are seen in nasal mucosa.[66]

CLINICAL APPLICATION AND GUIDELINES

Macrolide use in DPB and CF is well established, but other chronic inflammatory airway diseases are yet to have a macrolide-based treatment algorithm defined. Such was the response in DPB[1,4-7] that macrolide therapy has been applied to CF, chronic bronchitis, bronchiectasis, asthma, persistent rhinitis, and CRS. Perhaps too blunt an approach has been taken when managing many of these difficult-to-treat chronic pathologies. Asthma and CRS are potentially a heterogeneous group of pathologic mechanisms with a similar clinical presentation.[14,67-69] Based on current understanding of macrolide immunomodulation, it would seem unlikely that disease mechanisms dominated by eosinophilic and Th2 response will be macrolide sensitive.[47,70]

Clinical Use of Macrolides in Chronic Rhinosinusitis

Clinical effects appear to accompany reduction in proinflammatory cytokines in most CRS trials.[8] Only one randomized controlled trial has been performed to date[71] with an additional 11 nonplacebo controlled cohorts reported.[8] A summary of these trials is given in **Table 3**. Reduction of IL-8 dominates most of the objective outcomes.[71-73] Other cytokines, IL-6 and TNF-α, are also reduced in clinical trials.[72] Enhanced mucociliary function is reported.[62,74] Reduction of nasal polyps is often observed,[71,74,75] but the response is variable and often linked to smaller polyps. Only a few studies subclassify disease based on eosinophilia and systemic allergic response, which may explain the variable response. However, Ichimura and colleagues did not find an association of tissue eosinophilia and their response to treatment.[75]

Table 3
Clinical studies using macrolides

Type of Study	n	Dosage	Duration (Months)	Macrolide	Results	First Author of Study, Year
Prospective, double-blind, placebo controlled	64	150	3	RXM	Improvements in SNOT-20 score, nasal endoscopy, saccharine transit time, and IL-8 levels in lavage fluid (P<.05)	Wallwork, 2006
Prospective, randomized	90	1000 (2 wk), 500 (10 wk)	3	CAM	As effective as surgery in CRS	Ragab, 2004
Prospective, open	17	500	12	EM	12 responder, mucociliary, transport, headache, postnasal drip, all improved; P<.05	Cervin, 2002
Prospective, open	20	1000	0.5	CAM	Improvement in CD68, IL-6, IL-8, TNF-α, and clinical parameters	Macleod, 2001
Prospective, open	20	400	3	CAM	Reduction of IL-8 in nasal lavage, decreased nasal polyp size	Yamada, 2000
Prospective, open	16	200, 150	—	CAM, RXM	Patients with normal IgE had higher response rate	—
Prospective, open	20	1000	0, 5	CAM	Reduction of secretion volume, improvement in mucociliary transport	Rubin, 1997
Prospective, open	30	150	3	RXM	Approx. 80% of patients respond; postnasal drip, headache	Kimura, 1997
Prospective, open	12	150	—	RXM	Reduction of nasal IL-8, CT better aeration	Suzuki, 1997
Prospective, open	45	400	2–3	CAM	Approx. 71% overall improvement	Hashiba, 1996
Prospective, open	20 (+20 in combination with azelastine)	150	>2	RXM	Reduction of nasal polyps associated with CRS in at least 52% of patients	Ichimura, 1996
Prospective, open	32	400	1	CAM	Reduction of secretion volume, improvement in mucociliary transport	Nishi, 1995
Retrospective, open	149	200–600	3–6	EM	Postoperative treatment with EM improves results compared with no treatment, 88% improvement vs 68%	Moriyama, 1995
Prospective, open	16	600	>6	EM	Approx. 85% overall improvement	Iino, 1993
Prospective, open	?	400–600	8	EM	Approx. 60% overall improvement	Kikuchi, 1991

Full references are available in the source article.
Abbreviations: CAM, clarithromycin; EM, erythromycin; RXM, roxithromycin.
Data from Cervin A, Wallwork B. Anti-inflammatory effects of macrolide antibiotics in the treatment of chronic rhinosinusitis. Otolaryngol Clin North Am 2005;38:1339–50.

Table 4
Poor prognostic features for CRS response with low-dose macrolide therapy
Atopic predisposition
High serum IgE (>200–250 U/mL)
Response to effective distribution of topical steroid therapy
Watery discharge, itch- and sneeze-dominated symptomatology
Presence of asthma, dermatitis, or conjunctivitis
Ciliary disorders
Allergic fungal rhinosinusitis
No previous culture directed antibiotic therapy
Suspected eosinophilic inflammation

Duration of Therapy

Intracellular accumulation of macrolides, inhibition of transcription factors, and the suppression of cytokine production seem to take several weeks before an optimal clinical response is obtained. The impact of duration of therapy is significant for DPB. Macrolide therapy does not have a significant impact until 6 to 8 weeks into treatment. Response to therapy increased from 5% at 2 weeks to 71% at 12 weeks for DPB.[76] In the treatment of CRS, Hashiba and colleagues demonstrated time-dependent symptom relief in 71% of patients at 12 weeks.[76] This improvement increased rapidly after 6 to 8 weeks of therapy and possible continued improvement after 12 weeks. The double-blind, randomized controlled trial undertaken for macrolides in CRS showed a nonsignificant 6-week SNOT20 improvement that reached a mean decline of 0.32 ($P = .01$) at 12 weeks.[73] This result is less than the minimal clinical important difference for SNOT20. However, the "low IgE" groups fared significantly better, with a 0.70 ($P<.01$) difference at 12 weeks. Both improvements were lost at 3 months post therapy.

Prognostic Features Classification

There are good in vivo data and results from clinical trials[8] that suggest a strong predisposition to a neutrophilic immunomodulation by macrolides. Those pathologies that are dominated by eosinophilic mediated effector T-cell responses are less affected. The efficacy of low-dose macrolide antibiotic therapy is strongly influenced by the degree of Th2 skewed response.[70,73] Patients without atopy or eosinophilia are more likely to respond to either clarithromycin or roxithromycin. The presence of high IgE (>200–250 U/mL), peripheral eosinophilia, or nasal eosinophilia were poor prognostic factors (**Table 4**). Thus, those conditions in which these inflammatory mechanisms play a major role, such as allergic fungal rhinosinusitis, are unlikely to respond to macrolides. Unfortunately, the current classification system for chronic inflammatory rhinosinusitis is rudimentary, with only polyps and eosinophilic inflammation as the main subgroups. Allergic fungal rhinosinusitis, with its IgE-dominated etiology, is the only currently accepted additional category.[77]

SUMMARY

Suppression of neutrophilic inflammation of the airways has been demonstrated as the most robust immunomodulatory response from 14- and 15-membered ring macrolides. The inhibition of transcription factors, mainly NF-κB and AP-1, from alterations in intracellular cell signaling drive this mechanism. The suppression of IL-8 to a range of endogenous and exogenous challenges characterizes the effects on cytokine production. Evidence for a strong clinical effect in CRS is mounting, but results may be tempered by researchers' inability to characterize the disease process. Eosinophilia-dominated CRS is unlikely to respond, based on current research understanding and data from clinical trials.

REFERENCES

1. Kudoh S, Azuma A, Yamamoto M, et al. Improvement of survival in patients with diffuse panbronchiolitis treated with low-dose erythromycin. Am J Respir Crit Care Med 1998;157:1829–32.
2. Homma H, Yamanaka A, Tanimoto S, et al. Diffuse panbronchiolitis. A disease of the transitional zone of the lung. Chest 1983;83:63–9.
3. Sugiyama Y, Kudoh S, Maeda H, et al. Analysis of HLA antigens in patients with diffuse panbronchiolitis. Am Rev Respir Dis 1990;141:1459–62.
4. Kudoh S, Uetake T, Hagiwara M, et al. Clinical effect of low-dose long-term erythromycin chemotherapy on diffuse panbronchiolitis. Jpn J Thorac Dis 1987;25: 632–42.
5. Kadota J, Mukae H, Ishii H, et al. Long-term efficacy and safety of clarithromycin treatment in patients with diffuse panbronchiolitis. Respir Med 2003;97:844–50.
6. Nagai H, Shishido H, Yoneda R, et al. Long-term low-dose administration of erythromycin to patients with diffuse panbronchiolitis. Respiration 1991;58:145–9.
7. Kim YW, Park GY, Yoo CG, et al. Clinical effect of low-dose long-term erythromycin on diffuse panbronchiolitis. Tuberculosis and Respiratory Diseases 1994;41: 127–34.
8. Cervin A, Wallwork B. Macrolide therapy of chronic rhinosinusitis. Rhinology 2007; 45:259–67.
9. Robinson JA. Polyketide synthase complexes: their structure and function in antibiotic biosynthesis. Philos Trans R Soc Lond B Biol Sci 1991;332:107–44.
10. Omura S. Macrolide antibiotics: chemistry, biology, and practice. 2nd edition. Amsterdam; Boston: Academic Press; 2002.
11. Mascaretti OA. Bacteria versus antibacterial agents: an integrated approach. Washington, DC; [Great Britain]: ASM Press; 2003.
12. Farrell DJ, Morrissey I, Bakker S, et al. Molecular characterization of macrolide resistance mechanisms among Streptococcus pneumoniae and Streptococcus pyogenes isolated from the PROTEKT 1999–2000 study. J Antimicrob Chemother 2002;50(Suppl S1):39–47.
13. Hyde TB, Gay K, Stephens DS, et al. Macrolide resistance among invasive Streptococcus pneumoniae isolates. JAMA 2001;286:1857–62.
14. Fokkens W, Lund V, Mullol J, et al. European position paper on rhinosinusitis and nasal polyps 2007. Rhinology 2007;(Suppl 20):1–136.
15. Kern RC, Conley DB, Walsh W, et al. Perspectives on the etiology of chronic rhinosinusitis: an immune barrier hypothesis. Am J Rhinol 2008;22:549–59.
16. Lund VJ. Therapeutic targets in rhinosinusitis: infection or inflammation? Medscape J Med 2008;10:105.
17. Hatipoglu U, Rubinstein I. Anti-inflammatory treatment of chronic rhinosinusitis: a shifting paradigm. Curr Allergy Asthma Rep 2008;8:154–61.
18. Neuhaus O, Archelos JJ, Hartung HP. Immunomodulation in multiple sclerosis: from immunosuppression to neuroprotection. Trends Pharmacol Sci 2003;24:131–8.

19. Callard R, George AJ, Stark J. Cytokines, chaos, and complexity. Immunity 1999; 11:507–13.
20. Tamaoki J. The effects of macrolides on inflammatory cells. Chest 2004;125: 41S–50S, quiz 51S.
21. Stein GE, Havlichek DH. The new macrolide antibiotics. Azithromycin and clarithromycin. Postgrad Med 1992;92:269–72.
22. Bermudez LE, Inderlied C, Young LS. Stimulation with cytokines enhances penetration of azithromycin into human macrophages. Antimicrob Agents Chemother 1991;35:2625–9.
23. Cervin A, Wallwork B. Anti-inflammatory effects of macrolide antibiotics in the treatment of chronic rhinosinusitis. Otolaryngol Clin North Am 2005;38: 1339–50.
24. Fujii T, Kadota J, Kawakami K, et al. Long term effect of erythromycin therapy in patients with chronic *Pseudomonas aeruginosa* infection. Thorax 1995;50: 1246–52.
25. Kadota J, Sakito O, Kohno S, et al. A mechanism of erythromycin treatment in patients with diffuse panbronchiolitis. Am Rev Respir Dis 1993;147:153–9.
26. Sakito O, Kadota J, Kohno S, et al. Interleukin 1 beta, tumor necrosis factor alpha, and interleukin 8 in bronchoalveolar lavage fluid of patients with diffuse panbronchiolitis: a potential mechanism of macrolide therapy. Respiration 1996;63:42–8.
27. Tamaoki J, Kadota J, Takizawa H. Clinical implications of the immunomodulatory effects of macrolides. Am J Med 2004;117(Suppl 9A):5S–11S.
28. Tamaoki J, Takeyama K, Yamawaki I, et al. Lipopolysaccharide-induced goblet cell hypersecretion in the guinea pig trachea: inhibition by macrolides. Am J Phys 1997;272:L15–9.
29. Akamatsu H, Yamawaki M, Horio T. Effects of roxithromycin on adhesion molecules expressed on endothelial cells of the dermal microvasculature. J Int Med Res 2001;29:523–7.
30. Lin HC, Wang CH, Liu CY, et al. Erythromycin inhibits beta2-integrins (CD11b/CD18) expression, interleukin-8 release and intracellular oxidative metabolism in neutrophils. Respir Med 2000;94:654–60.
31. Matsuoka N, Eguchi K, Kawakami A, et al. Inhibitory effect of clarithromycin on costimulatory molecule expression and cytokine production by synovial fibroblast-like cells. Clin Exp Immunol 1996;104:501–8.
32. Abdelghaffar H, Vazifeh D, Labro MT. Erythromycin A-derived macrolides modify the functional activities of human neutrophils by altering the phospholipase D-phosphatidate phosphohydrolase transduction pathway: L-cladinose is involved both in alterations of neutrophil functions and modulation of this transductional pathway. J Immunol 1997;159:3995–4005.
33. Morikawa T, Kadota JI, Kohno S, et al. Superoxide dismutase in alveolar macrophages from patients with diffuse panbronchiolitis. Respiration 2000;67:546–51.
34. Levert H, Gressier B, Moutard I, et al. Azithromycin impact on neutrophil oxidative metabolism depends on exposure time. Inflammation 1998;22:191–201.
35. Bachert C, Wagenmann M, Rudack C, et al. The role of cytokines in infectious sinusitis and nasal polyposis. Allergy 1998;53:2–13.
36. Fujii T, Kadota J, Morikawa T, et al. Inhibitory effect of erythromycin on interleukin 8 production by 1 alpha, 25-dihydroxyvitamin D3-stimulated THP-1 cells. Antimicrob Agents Chemother 1996;40:1548–51.
37. Suzuki H, Asada Y, Ikeda K, et al. Inhibitory effect of erythromycin on interleukin-8 secretion from exudative cells in the nasal discharge of patients with chronic sinusitis. Laryngoscope 1999;109:407–10.

38. Kikuchi T, Hagiwara K, Honda Y, et al. Clarithromycin suppresses lipopolysaccha-ride-induced interleukin-8 production by human monocytes through AP-1 and NF-kappa B transcription factors. J Antimicrob Chemother 2002;49:745–55.
39. Desaki M, Takizawa H, Ohtoshi T, et al. Erythromycin suppresses nuclear factor-kappaB and activator protein-1 activation in human bronchial epithelial cells. Biochem Biophys Res Commun 2000;267:124–8.
40. Abe S, Nakamura H, Inoue S, et al. Interleukin-8 gene repression by clarithromycin is mediated by the activator protein-1 binding site in human bronchial epithelial cells. Am J Respir Cell Mol Biol 2000;22:51–60.
41. Desaki M, Okazaki H, Sunazuka T, et al. Molecular mechanisms of anti-inflamma-tory action of erythromycin in human bronchial epithelial cells: possible role in the signaling pathway that regulates nuclear factor-kappaB activation. Antimicrob Agents Chemother 2004;48:1581–5.
42. Shinkai M, Henke MO, Rubin BK. Macrolide antibiotics as immunomodulatory medications: proposed mechanisms of action. Pharmacol Ther 2008;117: 393–405.
43. Wallwork B, Coman W, Feron F, et al. Clarithromycin and prednisolone inhibit cytokine production in chronic rhinosinusitis. Laryngoscope 2002;112: 1827–30.
44. Wallwork B, Coman W, Mackay-Sim A, et al. Effect of clarithromycin on nuclear factor-kappa B and transforming growth factor-beta in chronic rhinosinusitis. Laryngoscope 2004;114:286–90.
45. Asano K, Kamakazu K, Hisamitsu T, et al. Modulation of Th2 type cytokine production from human peripheral blood leukocytes by a macrolide antibiotic, roxithromycin, in vitro. Int Immunopharmacol 2001;1:1913–21.
46. Morikawa K, Zhang J, Nonaka M, et al. Modulatory effect of macrolide antibi-otics on the Th1- and Th2-type cytokine production. Int J Antimicrob Agents 2002;19:53–9.
47. Wallwork B, Coman W. Chronic rhinosinusitis and eosinophils: do macrolides have an effect? Curr Opin Otolaryngol Head Neck Surg 2004;12:14–7.
48. Tamaoki J, Kondo M, Kohri K, et al. Macrolide antibiotics protect against immune complex-induced lung injury in rats: role of nitric oxide from alveolar macro-phages. J Immunol 1999;163:2909–15.
49. Oda H, Kadota J, Kohno S, et al. Leukotriene B4 in bronchoalveolar lavage fluid of patients with diffuse panbronchiolitis. Chest 1995;108:116–22.
50. Hirakata Y, Kaku M, Mizukane R, et al. Potential effects of erythromycin on host defense systems and virulence of Pseudomonas aeruginosa. Antimicrob Agents Chemother 1992;36:1922–7.
51. Baumann U, Fischer JJ, Gudowius P, et al. Buccal adherence of Pseudomonas aeruginosa in patients with cystic fibrosis under long-term therapy with azithro-mycin. Infection 2001;29:7–11.
52. Tsang KW, Ng P, Ho PL, et al. Effects of erythromycin on Pseudomonas aeruginosa adherence to collagen and morphology in vitro. Eur Respir J 2003;21:401–6.
53. Wozniak DJ, Keyser R. Effects of subinhibitory concentrations of macrolide antibiotics on Pseudomonas aeruginosa. Chest 2004;125:62S–9S, quiz 69S.
54. Nalca Y, Jansch L, Bredenbruch F, et al. Quorum-sensing antagonistic activities of azithromycin in Pseudomonas aeruginosa PAO1: a global approach. Antimicrob Agents Chemother 2006;50:1680–8.
55. Sofer D, Gilboa-Garber N, Belz A, et al. 'Subinhibitory' erythromycin represses production of Pseudomonas aeruginosa lectins, autoinducer and virulence factors. Chemotherapy 1999;45:335–41.

56. Mitsuya Y, Kawai S, Kobayashi H. Influence of macrolides on guanosine diphospho-D-mannose dehydrogenase activity in *Pseudomonas* biofilm. J Infect Chemother 2000;6:45–50.

57. Takeoka K, Ichimiya T, Yamasaki T, et al. The in vitro effect of macrolides on the interaction of human polymorphonuclear leukocytes with *Pseudomonas aeruginosa* in biofilm. Chemotherapy 1998;44:190–7.

58. Yanagihara K, Tomono K, Imamura Y, et al. Effect of clarithromycin on chronic respiratory infection caused by *Pseudomonas aeruginosa* with biofilm formation in an experimental murine model. J Antimicrob Chemother 2002;49:867–70.

59. Tamaoki J, Nakata J, Tagaya E, et al. Effects of roxithromycin and erythromycin on interleukin 8-induced neutrophil recruitment and goblet cell secretion in guinea pig tracheas. Antimicrob Agents Chemother 1996;40:1726–8.

60. Tamaoki J, Takeyama K, Tagaya E, et al. Effect of clarithromycin on sputum production and its rheological properties in chronic respiratory tract infections. Antimicrob Agents Chemother 1995;39:1688–90.

61. Rhee CS, Majima Y, Arima S, et al. Effects of clarithromycin on rheological properties of nasal mucus in patients with chronic sinusitis. Ann Otol Rhinol Laryngol 2000;109:484–7.

62. Nishi K, Mizuguchi M, Tachibana H, et al. Effect of clarithromycin on symptoms and mucociliary transport in patients with sino-bronchial syndrome. Nihon Kyobu Shikkan Gakkai Zasshi. Japanese J Thorac Dis 1995;33:1392–400.

63. Tagaya E, Tamaoki J, Kondo M, et al. Effect of a short course of clarithromycin therapy on sputum production in patients with chronic airway hypersecretion. Chest 2002;122:213–8.

64. Ikeda K, Wu D, Takasaka T. Inhibition of acetylcholine-evoked Cl^- currents by 14-membered macrolide antibiotics in isolated acinar cells of the guinea pig nasal gland. Am J Respir Cell Mol Biol 1995;13:449–54.

65. Rubin BK. Physiology of airway mucus clearance. Respir Care 2002;47:761–8.

66. Shimizu T, Shimizu S, Hattori R, et al. In vivo and in vitro effects of macrolide antibiotics on mucus secretion in airway epithelial cells. Am J Respir Crit Care Med 2003;168:581–7.

67. Simpson JL, Scott R, Boyle MJ, et al. Inflammatory subtypes in asthma: assessment and identification using induced sputum. Respirology 2006;11:54–61.

68. Ferguson BJ. Clarification of terminology in patients with eosinophilic and noneosinophilic hyperplastic rhinosinusitis [comment]. J Allergy Clin Immunol 2003;112:221–2, author reply 222–3.

69. Ferguson BJ. Categorization of eosinophilic chronic rhinosinusitis. Curr Opin Otolaryngol Head Neck Surg 2004;12:237–42.

70. Suzuki H, Ikeda K, Honma R, et al. Prognostic factors of chronic rhinosinusitis under long-term low-dose macrolide therapy. ORL J Otorhinolaryngol Relat Spec 2000;62:121–7.

71. Wallwork B, Coman W, Mackay-Sim A, et al. A double-blind, randomized, placebo-controlled trial of macrolide in the treatment of chronic rhinosinusitis. Laryngoscope 2006;116:189–93.

72. MacLeod CM, Hamid QA, Cameron L, et al. Anti-inflammatory activity of clarithromycin in adults with chronically inflamed sinus mucosa. Adv Ther 2001;18:75–82.

73. Yamada T, Fujieda S, Mori S, et al. Macrolide treatment decreased the size of nasal polyps and IL-8 levels in nasal lavage. Am J Rhinol 2000;14:143–8.

74. Ragab SM, Lund VJ, Scadding G. Evaluation of the medical and surgical treatment of chronic rhinosinusitis: a prospective, randomised, controlled trial. Laryngoscope 2004;114:923–30.

75. Ichimura K, Shimazaki Y, Ishibashi T, et al. Effect of new macrolide roxithromycin upon nasal polyps associated with chronic sinusitis. Auris Nasus Larynx 1996;23: 48–56.

76. Hashiba M, Baba S. Efficacy of long-term administration of clarithromycin in the treatment of intractable chronic sinusitis. Supplement. Acta Otolaryngol 1996; 525:73–8.

77. Meltzer EO, Hamilos DL, Hadley JA, et al. Rhinosinusitis: developing guidance for clinical trials. Otolaryngol Head Neck Surg 2006;135:S31–80.

78. Hoffmann N, Lee B, Hentzer M, et al. Azithromycin blocks quorum sensing and alginate polymer formation and increases the sensitivity to serum and stationary-growth-phase killing of *Pseudomonas aeruginosa* and attenuates chronic *P aeruginosa* lung infection in Cftr(-/-) mice. Antimicrob Agents Chemother 2007;51:3677–87.

79. Gillis RJ, Iglewski BH. Azithromycin retards Pseudomonas aeruginosa biofilm formation. J Clin Microbiol 2004;42:5842–5.

80. Imamura Y, Yanagihara K, Mizuta Y, et al. Azithromycin inhibits MUC5AC production induced by the Pseudomonas aeruginosa autoinducer N-(3-Oxododecanoyl) homoserine lactone in NCI-H292 Cells. Antimicrob Agents Chemother 2004;48: 3457–61.

81. Carter G, Young LS, Bermudez LE. A subinhibitory concentration of clarithromycin inhibits Mycobacterium avium biofilm formation. Antimicrob Agents Chemother 2004;48:4907–10.

82. Favre-Bonte S, Kohler T, Van Delden C. Biofilm formation by *Pseudomonas aeruginosa*: role of the C4-HSL cell-to-cell signal and inhibition by azithromycin. J Antimicrob Chemother 2003;52:598–604.

83. Tateda K, Comte R, Pechere JC, et al. Azithromycin inhibits quorum sensing in *Pseudomonas aeruginosa*. Antimicrob Agents Chemother 2001;45:1930–3.

84. Kawamura-Sato K, Iinuma Y, Hasegawa T, et al. Effect of subinhibitory concentrations of macrolides on expression of flagellin in *Pseudomonas aeruginosa* and Proteus mirabilis. Antimicrob Agents Chemother 2000;44:2869–72.

85. Tateda K, Ishii Y, Matsumoto T, et al. Potential of macrolide antibiotics to inhibit protein synthesis of *Pseudomonas aeruginosa*: suppression of virulence factors and stress response. J Infect Chemother 2000;6:1–7.

86. Ichimiya T, Takeoka K, Hiramatsu K, et al. The influence of azithromycin on the biofilm formation of *Pseudomonas aeruginosa* in vitro. Chemother 1996;42: 186–91.

87. Mizukane R, Hirakata Y, Kaku M, et al. Comparative in vitro exoenzyme-suppressing activities of azithromycin and other macrolide antibiotics against *Pseudomonas aeruginosa*. Antimicrob Agents Chemother 1994;38:528–33.

88. Yasuda H, Ajiki Y, Koga T, et al. Interaction between clarithromycin and biofilms formed by *Staphylococcus epidermidis*. Antimicrob Agents Chemother 1994; 38:138–41.

Chronic Rhinosinusitis in Children: What are the Treatment Options?

Arthur W. Wu, MD[a], Nina L. Shapiro, MD[a], Neil Bhattacharyya, MD[b],*

KEYWORDS

- Chronic rhinosinusitis • Pediatrics • Antibiotics
- Adenoidectomy • Therapy

Rhinosinusitis is one of the most common health problems in the United States and affects approximately 31 million Americans annually.[1] In adults, quality-of-life surveys have shown that the effects of sinusitis on Americans are comparable to those of diabetes or congestive heart failure.[2] The effect on quality of life for chronic rhinosinusitis (CRS) in the pediatric population is also significant.[3] Since this group is prone to frequent upper respiratory tract infections, the diagnosis of CRS can be more difficult to make. The prevalence of CRS in the pediatric population is inversely related to the age of the patient, and younger age groups have higher incidences of both viral upper respiratory infections (URIs) and CRS.[4] Indeed, CRS may lie within a spectrum of disorders with similar presenting symptoms like those of viral upper respiratory tract infections or allergic rhinitis.

DIAGNOSIS

Diagnosing CRS in children can be more difficult than diagnosing CRS in adults, as a physician must determine whether the pediatric patient truly has CRS or merely has frequent upper respiratory tract infections, perennial allergic rhinitis, or other similar disorders. The diagnosis of pediatric CRS is based on guidelines originally laid out for diagnosing CRS in adults. The Rhinosinusitis Task Force in 1996 and the Task Force for Defining Adult Chronic Rhinosinusitis in 2003 included experts from multiple disciplines to provide a consensus definition and method for diagnosing CRS. They recommended the diagnosis of CRS be made in those patients who demonstrate common CRS-associated symptoms (two major symptoms or one major with two minor symptoms) for 12 weeks or more and who have either radiographic or endoscopic evidence supporting the diagnosis.[5,6]

[a] Division of Otolaryngology, Department of Surgery, David Geffen School of Medicine at UCLA, 62-158 CHS, 10833 Leconte Avenue, Los Angeles, CA 90095, USA
[b] Division of Otolaryngology, Department of Otology & Laryngology, Brigham and Women's Hospital, Harvard Medical School, 45 Francis Street, Boston, MA 02115, USA
* Corresponding author.
E-mail address: neiloy@massmed.org (N. Bhattacharyya).

Immunol Allergy Clin N Am 29 (2009) 705–717
doi:10.1016/j.iac.2009.07.007   immunology.theclinics.com

The symptoms of CRS in children may be different from those in adults and the manifestations of these symptoms can also be age dependent. For example, facial pain in an infant may only manifest itself as irritability. Chronic cough, however, does seem to be a very common problem and presenting symptom in pediatric patients with CRS.[7] Objective symptoms witnessed by parents, such as cough, nasal discharge, or nasal obstruction, may be more reliable in younger children. In younger patients, parents often must act as the proxy for describing their child's sinus symptoms. However, older children and adolescents may be more descriptive in evaluating their own health and are able to describe more localized symptoms, such as nasal congestion, otalgia, facial pressure/pain, or hyposmia.

Children are less tolerant to outpatient endoscopic examination of the sinuses, but using appropriately sized flexible endoscopes or traditional anterior rhinoscopy with an otoscope or mirror can usually add critical information regarding the inflammatory status of the nasal cavity. The radiologic study of choice in diagnosing CRS is CT; only 2% of practicing otolaryngologists in a recent study use plain radiographs as their study of choice.[8] Plain radiographs tend to be less reliable and may overcall the amount of mucosal thickening, depending on the angle of exposure. Several studies have demonstrated that CT scans have excellent sensitivity and specificity for diagnosing CRS in children. Unlike adults, where a normal Lund-McKay score should be 0, in children without CRS is about 3, and the diagnostic cutoff for an abnormal CT is a score of 5 or above.[9,10] While CT scans are more accurate, they also expose the pediatric patient to radiation, which may increase the risk of developing future malignancies. This risk should be well considered before ordering a CT scan if diagnosis can be achieved without radiologic confirmation.

PATHOGENESIS

Understanding the pathogenesis of CRS is critical in its management. The difficulty lies in determining the exact factors that have contributed to creating chronic sinusitis in a specific patient. The etiology of chronic rhinosinusitis is not completely understood but derives from interactions among local host factors, systemic host factors, and environmental factors. The treatment options for pediatric chronic rhinosinusitis are aimed at treating these different etiologies.

Local host factors, such as anatomic abnormalities, are uncommon in children.[11] However, if physical examination and radiology suggest structural anomalies, such as septal deviation, concha bullosa, or Haller cells, then this information may drive the treatment course toward surgery. Obstruction of nasal drainage pathways by enlarged adenoids was once thought to be a causative factor in CRS.[12] However, recent studies have shown no relation between large adenoids and increased incidence of CRS.[13–16]

Systemic host factors, such as allergies, gastroesophageal reflux disease (GERD), and mucociliary dysfunction, also play a role in the pathogenesis of CRS. Allergy and asthma have been implicated to have a large role in the pathogenesis of CRS. Early reports suggested that up to 70% of children with CRS also have allergic rhinitis, a higher incidence than in the general population.[17,18] Childhood asthmatics are also predisposed to CRS.[19] Some reports demonstrate a predisposing role for allergy and asthma in the pathogenesis of CRS. Those patients with nasal polyposis have an additional causal mechanism for CRS from the anatomic blockage of their natural drainage pathways. In contrast, however, some recent studies, including the Italian arm of the International Study on Allergies and Asthma in Childhood (ISAAC) study, have shown an incidence of allergies in pediatric CRS patients similar to that of the general population, approximately 30%.[20,21]

Despite the unclear causal relationship between allergy, asthma, and CRS, it has become commonly accepted that there is likely a connection between these conditions. According to the "united airway theory," allergic rhinitis, asthma, and CRS are all manifestations of inflammation of a continuous airway and lie on a spectrum of symptoms rather than define distinct disease entities. Exacerbations of inflammation of the lower respiratory tract can compromise the upper respiratory tract, and the reverse also holds true.[22] Several studies have demonstrated that the mucosa in pediatric CRS shows increased eosinophils and lymphocytes compared with normal mucosa.[23,24] However, CRS in children may be a slightly different disease than that in adults as the inflammatory infiltrate shows more neutrophils and lymphocytes with fewer eosinophils.[25]

GERD is another systemic host factor that has been implicated as a cause of local inflammation and as a predisposing factor in CRS.[26,27] Incidence of GERD may be higher in infants than in the adult population. With GERD, the nasopharynx and nasal cavity is washed with gastric contents, which may cause the mucosa to undergo chronic inflammatory changes, resulting in CRS.[28] A study by Phipps[29] demonstrated a high prevalence of GERD (63%) in pediatric patients with medically refractory CRS based on upper esophageal and nasopharyngeal pH probes.

Children with impaired mucociliary clearance, such as children with cystic fibrosis or, less commonly, primary ciliary dyskinesia or Kartagener disease, are at high risk for chronic sinusitis. CRS in these patients is difficult to manage, and such patients may benefit from more prompt surgical intervention and aggressive irrigation. Ciliary dysfunction can be diagnosed with nasal or tracheal mucosal biopsies. Diagnosis of cystic fibrosis involves the sweat chloride test or, more recently, genetic testing. Cystic fibrosis can result from any one of a plethora of different mutations in the cystic fibrosis transmembrane regulator gene (CFTR), which is a gene for a membrane chloride channel. The specific mutation or genotype leads to varying degrees of severity of disease in these patients. Specifically, those with complete absence of this protein channel have more acute and severe rhinosinusitis, while those with milder mutations with partially functional chloride channels are more likely to have CRS.[30]

Environmental factors, such as infectious microorgansims and noxious inhalants, may also contribute in the development of CRS. As previously mentioned, adenoid size does not seem to correlate with CRS in children, but the adenoid itself may still play a role in CRS as a reservoir of pathogenic bacteria. When mucociliary clearance is compromised during URI or in allergic rhinitis, bacteria may gain access to the sinus and nasal cavity and initiate sinusitis. Studies have demonstrated that sinonasal symptoms correlate with the quantity of bacterial colonization in the adenoids.[31,32] Additionally, bacterial cultures taken from both the lateral nasal wall and the adenoids in individual patients with CRS demonstrate identical strains of bacteria, lending support to the notion that the adenoids may act as a source of bacteria that become pathogenic in CRS.[33] The adenoids in children with CRS have also been shown to be covered with a biofilm of bacteria.[34] Biofilms are resistant to antibiotics and may provide a reservoir of bacteria in patients with CRS. Clearing the nasal cavity and sinuses of this source of bacteria is the reasoning behind performing adenoidectomy in children with CRS.

Inhaled pollutants can irritate the upper aerodigestive tract, including the nose and sinus cavities. The most common pollutant and most significant is tobacco smoke, which has been shown to be a poor prognostic indicator in CRS.[35] Possible reasons for this include cigarette smoke's inhibition of mucociliary clearance and epithelial regeneration.[36]

TREATMENT OVERVIEW

The treatment of CRS in children is divided between medical and surgical management. Initial treatment of pediatric CRS should be medical except in those cases where there is obvious anatomic obstruction. Children with cystic fibrosis or mucociliary dyskinesis may also need to be treated more aggressively. Additionally, the dictum of preserving natural drainage pathways may not apply in these patients. Gravity-based drainage may be more effective.

Medical Therapy

Medical treatment of CRS should, at the very least, treat both infection and inflammation. This is supported by a relatively recent outcome-based clinical practice guideline that recommended a combination of an antibiotic and a nasal steroid spray.[37] However, these guidelines did not make any specific recommendations for the duration of antibiotic treatment. Short-term antibiotic treatment of CRS has been shown to be inadequate to relieve symptoms.[38,39] Despite lack of long-term outcome data, most recommend duration of treatment from 3 to 6 weeks.[40–42] Resistance to long-term antibiotic treatment is a good indicator that surgical intervention may be warranted.

In addition to the duration of treatment, the choice of antibiotic is also important and must take into account the polymicrobial nature of infection in CRS as well as common resistance patterns. Typically, patients with CRS have undergone multiple courses of antibiotics, and the prevalence of antibiotic-resistant pathogens is quite high. One study demonstrated 72% of *Streptococcus pneumoniae*, 60% of *Haemophilus influenzae*, and 58% of *Moraxella catarrhalis* isolated from the middle meatus of children with rhinosinusitis were resistant to first-line antibiotics.[43] Ideally, the choice of antibiotic is based on culture susceptibility results. However, CRS often presents without frank purulent material to be cultured, and reliable culture results may require tissue, which is not an option in the outpatient clinical setting. More sensitive testing methods in the future, such as polymerase chain reaction, may lead to more accurate culture results and may help with focusing antibiotic therapy toward specific pathogens.[44] While there is no consensus recommendation for a single first-line antibiotic in CRS,[42,45] we recommend a broad-spectrum agent be used, such as amoxicillin-clavulanic acid. If methicillin-resistant *Staphylococcus aureus* is suspected, a combination of clindamycin and trimethoprim-sulfamethoxazole is an option. In those patients with cystic fibrosis, fluoroquinolones may be considered because of the high incidence of *Pseudomonas aeruginosa* in these patients. In the adult population, there has been evidence that macrolide antibiotics may be beneficial in the treatment of CRS. Several studies have demonstrated that macrolides may have anti-inflammatory effects in addition to their bacteriostatic primary function.[46–49] Unfortunately, there have not been similar studies focusing on pediatric patients, but future studies may extrapolate these results to children with CRS.

Similar to long-term oral macrolide therapy, long-term intravenous antibiotics may also treat the low-level underlying infection and osteitis more effectively than a short course of oral antibiotics. One retrospective study evaluated the efficacy of intravenous antibiotic treatment alone for CRS and found it to be efficacious in 22 of 22 patients (100%) with approximately 70% of patients deriving long-term benefits from this treatment alone. While the cost of such treatment is quite significant, the investigators note that it is still significantly less than the cost of a typical functional endoscopic sinus surgery (FESS).[50]

The role of fungal infection in CRS is currently a contentious subject.[51] While several studies have shown the presence of fungus in patients with CRS, the clinical significance of this remains unclear, as fungal colonization is common in the general population as well.[52] Some proponents of a fungal etiology of CRS have proposed topical amphotericin B as a possible treatment for CRS. The data supporting this theory are minimal with only a few studies showing any benefit. Ponikau and colleagues[53] have shown subjective improvement in 75% of adult patients, with objective improvement in endoscopic examination. A randomized, placebo-controlled, double-blind trial by the same group found reduced mucosal thickening on CT and endoscopy but no difference in symptoms.[54] Several adult studies attempting to repeat these results showed no changes after treatment.[55,56,57] There have been no studies in the pediatric population regarding the efficacy of amphotericin B nasal irrigation. Additionally, compliance with nasal irrigation of any kind is difficult in the pediatric setting because of patient intolerance. The future testing of this hypothesis may include oral antifungals, which would be more feasible in the pediatric population. Until then, the use of antifungals in pediatric CRS cannot be broadly recommended.

In addition to antimicrobials, medical therapy should include the use of nasal steroid spray.[42] While there are no randomized clinical trials supporting this recommendation, decreasing the inflammation inherent to this disease is beneficial. According to the "united airway theory," the upper and lower airways are not independent entities, and inflammatory diseases, such as allergic rhinitis, asthma, and CRS, affect the entire airway. Patients with concomitant allergic rhinitis and asthma may exacerbate their sinonasal symptoms with reduced mucociliary clearance and increased inflammation. Additionally, it has been clearly documented that CRS can exacerbate asthma. Treatment of CRS leads to a reduction in asthma attacks and can actually change the inflammatory milieu in these patients.[58–60] However, there is a dearth of clinical studies evaluating the use of intranasal steroids for all children with CRS. The widespread use of intranasal steroids for CRS is mostly anecdotal. A review of the literature concluded a probable, modest benefit from topical intranasal steroid use.[61] Recent surveys of practicing otolaryngologists reported that approximately 90% use nasal steroid sprays together with oral antibiotics to manage pediatric CRS.[8,62] Currently, mometasone furoate is the only intranasal steroid spray approved for children older than 2 years of age. Long-term studies show no effect on growth or the pituitary axis.[63,64] Fluticasone propionate has been approved for children older than 4 years of age.

While adjunctive therapies, such as oral antihistamines, nasal saline irrigation, short-term oral steroids, and mucolytic agents, do not have much support in the scientific literature, their use may provide symptomatic relief without many side effects. When intranasal steroids fail to relieve mucosal inflammation or nasal polyps, a short oral steroid course can be beneficial.[65] A recent study in adults showed that the use of baby shampoo irrigations as a topical mucolytic agent resulted in the majority of patients experiencing decreased symptoms of thickened mucus with approximately 40% experiencing overall improvement in their CRS-related symptoms.[66] As previously mentioned, compliance with irrigations may be difficult in some pediatric patients, and oral mucolytics, such as guaifenesin, may be more tolerable. However, there are no studies testing its efficacy in children with CRS. We suggest that "maximal medical therapy" for pediatric CRS should include extended use of a broad-spectrum antibiotic and nasal steroid spray with or without adjunctive use of an oral antihistamine, an oral mucolytic agent, oral steroids, or nasal saline irrigation.

Before considering surgery, other conditions exacerbating the patient's sinonasal pathology need to be determined. Phipps[29] found that approximately 60% of pediatric patients who failed medical treatment of CRS suffered from GERD. Antireflux therapy significantly improved sinonasal symptoms in approximately 80% of this group. Other less-common disorders, such as cystic fibrosis, immunodeficiency, and primary ciliary dsykinesia, must also be considered if a child with CRS fails medical treatment. Primary ciliary dyskinesia and Kartagener syndrome can be diagnosed with nasal mucosal biopsies. While there is no medical treatment specifically for these disorders, diagnosis may lead to earlier initiation of maximal medical therapy, chronic preventative antibiotic use, or surgical intervention.

Chronic exposure to inhaled pollutants may prevent efficacy of medical treatment of CRS. Children living in homes with parents who are smokers may also have a poor outcome after medical or surgical treatment,[35] and such parents should be strongly encouraged to cease smoking or eliminate the child's exposure to noxious inhalants.

Surgical Therapy

Surgery is indicated in children who have failed "maximal medical therapy" and should be provided in a stepwise fashion. Adenoidectomy is the first-line surgical therapy in most children with CRS. Those who do not have a clinically significant adenoid pad or fail adenoidectomy should be considered for FESS.[28,41,67]

Adenoidectomy

There is evidence that the adenoid provides a reservoir of bacteria that may be a pathogenic factor in the development of CRS in children.[31–33] Biofilms overlying the adenoid pad may prevent antibiotic therapy from clearing the infection.[34] Adenoidectomy surgically removes this reservoir for chronic infection. Many studies have shown the efficacy and safety of adenoidectomy in children with CRS. The efficacy of adenoidectomy in alleviating sinonasal symptoms in these studies range from 50% to 70%.[41,67–70] While the relatively high cure rates from such studies are encouraging, symptoms of a significant number of patients are not relieved by adenoidectomy alone, which supports a multifactorial etiology of CRS in children. It would be beneficial to group patients by their probability of success with adenoidectomy to avoid unnecessary interventions or to know when to be more aggressive surgically. Ramadan[70] showed that patients with asthma or with a high Lund-McKay CT score are less likely to derive benefit from adenoidectomy alone. Therefore, these patients may benefit from an adenoidectomy combined with FESS for optimal primary surgical treatment.

Adenoidectomy with antral lavage

Several studies have attempted to optimize the benefit of adenoidectomy by adding adjunctive treatments at the time of surgery or during the postoperative period. Several investigators have used the opportunity of their patient being under general anesthesia to also perform maxillary sinus lavage. The lavage is used to both clear secretions and infection in the sinuses as well as to provide culture material to direct postoperative antibiotic therapy. Two of these studies combined adenoidectomy with maxillary sinus lavage and long-term intravenous antibiotic treatment.[71,72] The rate of resolution of symptoms after this treatment regimen was close to 80%, much higher than the rate reported with adenoidectomy alone. Drawbacks to long-term intravenous antibiotics are associated thrombophlebitis (one requiring venotomy in this study), pseudomembranous colitis, serum sickness, and drug fevers.[72]

While there seems to be some added benefit from intravenous antibiotic treatment, Ramadan[73] showed similar rates of symptom improvement (88%) with adenoidectomy and maxillary sinus lavage alone, without intravenous antibiotics. The cost of adding a simple lavage to an adenoidectomy in terms of time and resources are minimal. Such adjunctive procedures at the time of adenoidectomy or afterwards appear to be both efficacious and cost-effective.

Functional endoscopic sinus surgery

When adenoidectomy fails, FESS is the next step in surgical intervention for CRS. Additionally, patients without enlarged adenoids or patients with disorders affecting mucociliary clearance, such as cystic fibrosis or Kartagener syndrome, can be offered FESS as a first surgical option. FESS has been shown to be an extremely successful treatment of CRS in the adult population.[74] The adoption of FESS in children has been far less widespread, mainly because of concerns of hindering midface growth.[75] While this prejudice may still linger, the theory has been refuted by several large studies.[76,77] Bothwell and colleagues[77] evaluated patients over a 10-year period and found no difference in facial growth when comparing patients who underwent FESS and those who did not.

FESS differs from older forms of sinus surgery in that it focuses on preserving physiologic drainage pathways by enlarging the natural ostia.[78] The outcomes of FESS in children are excellent, with symptom improvement ranging from 80% to 100%.[79,80] Risks include injury to the globe, cerebrospinal fluid leak, nasolacrimal duct injury, and bleeding, but the overall complication rate is very low. A recent meta-analysis demonstrated a major complication rate of 0.6% with only 4 major complications reported from 690 FESS cases (2 cases of meningitis, 2 cases of intra-operative hemorrhage requiring transfusion).[80] Regardless, the treatment of CRS with FESS in children should be conservative; the literature recommends that initially only a maxillary antrostomy and anterior ethmoidectomy should be performed.[8] This treatment has been shown to be sufficient in most cases of CRS. Preoperative assessment before FESS in children is essential and includes a CT scan to delineate the anatomy of the sinuses. This is especially important in the pediatric population as the sinuses themselves are smaller (or sometimes absent) and can change in appearance and size with a child's growth. Anatomic abnormalities, such as a deviated septum or a concha bullosa, must be identified preoperatively or FESS failure may result without proper treatment of these conditions.

The postoperative care of pediatric FESS patients is important, and patients should remain on "maximal medical therapy" for several weeks after surgery. Saline irrigation is also ideal but may be difficult in the pediatric population. Adult patients may need to have extensive sinus cavity debridements in the outpatient setting postoperatively. These are almost impossible to accomplish in children. Second-look endoscopy was initially widely accepted as necessary for good outcomes in pediatric FESS.[81] However, this paradigm has shifted, and the majority of otolaryngologists currently do not endorse a second look. Second-look endoscopy does not seem to affect clinical outcome and exposes the patient to another general anesthesic.[82]

While both adenoidectomy and FESS have been shown to be effective treatments for CRS, the clinician should properly inform the patient and parents to expect significant symptom improvement but not an absolute cure. While it is possible that FESS may have a higher rate of success than adenoidectomy,[41] a stepwise approach in the surgical treatment is recommended. Adenoidectomy is a low-risk procedure, can be performed by almost all otolaryngologists, and has been shown to have substantial benefits in children with CRS. Alternatively, FESS in the pediatric population is technically more difficult, and surgery should only be performed with those with significant experience in FESS in children or with pediatric- and rhinology-trained otolaryngologists. A recent retrospective analysis on image guidance used in pediatric FESS demonstrated that this technology may be helpful for complicated cases involving the frontal sinus, sphenoid sinus, orbit, or skull base.[83]

Surgery in selected populations

As previously mentioned, there are populations of patients where it is appropriate for surgeons to intervene sooner in the treatment of CRS. Patients with ciliary dyskinesia, cystic fibrosis, allergic fungal sinusitis, or compromised immune systems benefit from prompt surgical management. CRS in these patients is difficult to treat, and these patients frequently require revision surgery.[84]

Primary ciliary dyskinesia and Kartagener syndrome are rare disorders resulting in chronic upper and lower airway infections. FESS has been shown to be effective in the management of CRS in these patients in case series, but no large group data exists because of the rarity of these disorders.[85] Patients with cystic fibrosis often have diffuse nasal polyposis and chronically infected sinuses with thick drainage. Aggressive surgical therapy has been shown to have long-term benefit for these patients, even though revision surgery and polyp regrowth is commonplace.[86] In patients with cystic fibrosis or ciliary dyskinesia, the etiology of CRS lies in the inability of mucus clearance via the natural sinus ostia, and surgeries providing gravity-based drainage, such as the mega-antrostomy, may benefit these patients.[87]

CRS can be a difficult problem in those patients with immunodeficiency, as the patient does not have a normal immune system to combat bacterial or fungal pathogens. Rhinosinusitis is one of the most common complications of primary humoral immunodeficiency, and primary immunodeficiency may be relatively common in patients with refractory CRS.[87,88] Patients with HIV/AIDS or those with chemotherapy-compromised immune systems are susceptible to opportunistic infections and may be more susceptible to severe complications from rhinosinusitis, such as abscess, meningitis, or venous thrombosis, among others. Because of the risk of these more serious complications, FESS should be offered in an acute setting should appropriate medical therapy, such as intravenous antibiotics, fail. Additionally, with improvements in HIV treatment extending the lives of HIV patients, CRS has been recognized to affect a large number of HIV-positive patients and diminish their quality of life. FESS has been demonstrated to alleviate symptoms and benefit the quality of life in these patients.[89]

Allergic fungal sinusitis may occur in the pediatric population and present with nasal symptoms, atopy, headaches, and ocular symptoms. The literature suggests that proptosis may be more common in children with allergic fungal sinusitis than in adults or young adults.[90] FESS should be offered to patients suspected of having allergic fungal sinusitis as the allergic mucin in the sinuses is thick and not easily cleared. These patients have a high relapse rate and should also be maintained postoperatively on maximal medical therapy, including sinus irrigation and nasal steroids. Additionally, patients with allergic fungal sinusitis should undergo immunotherapy for allergy to fungi.[90]

SUMMARY

The treatment of CRS in children relies on an understanding of the pathogenesis of the disease and proper diagnosis. The vast majority of patients should be initially managed with medical therapy. When "maximal medical therapy" fails, surgical intervention should be considered. Both adenoidectomy and FESS have been shown to be effective and safe in the pediatric population. Adenoidectomy should be considered as the first-line surgical treatment in all except those without significant adenoids, those with clear anatomic abnormalities causing CRS, or those with abnormal muco-ciliary clearance. This approach to the treatment of children with CRS will improve the symptoms and quality of life in the majority of patients.

REFERENCES

1. Slavin RG. Management of sinusitis. J Am Geriatr Soc 1991;39:212–7.
2. Gliklich RE, Metson R. The health impact of chronic sinusitis in patients seeking otolaryngologic care. Otolaryngol Head Neck Surg 1995;113:104–9.
3. Cunninham MJ, Chiu EJ, Landgraf JM, et al. The health impact of chronic rhino-sinusitis in children. Arch Otolaryngol Head Neck Surg 2000;126:1363–8.
4. Nguyen KL, Corbett ML, Garcia DP, et al. Chronic sinusitis among pediatric patients with chronic respiratory complaints. J Allergy Clin Immunol 1993;92: 824–30.
5. Lanza DC, Kennedy DW. Adult rhinosinusitis defined. Otolaryngol Head Neck Surg 1997;117(3:2):S1–7.
6. Benninger MS, Ferguson BJ, Hadley JA, et al. Adult chronic rhinosinusitis: defini-tions, diagnosis, epidemiology, and pathophysiology. Otolaryngol Head Neck Surg 2003;129(3):S1–32.
7. Wald ER. Management of sinusitis in infants and children. Pediatr Infect Dis J 1988;7:449–52.
8. Sobol SE, Samadi DS, Kazahaya K, et al. Trends in the management of chronic sinusitis: a survey of the American Society of Pediatric Otolaryngology. Laryngo-scope 2005;115:78–80.
9. Bhattacharyya N, Jones DT, Hill M, et al. The diagnostic accuracy of computed tomography in pediatric chronic rhinosinusitis. Arch Otolaryngol Head Neck Surg 2004;130(9):1029–32.
10. Hill M, Bhattacharyya N, Hall TR, et al. Incidental paranasal sinus imaging abnor-malities and the normal Lund score in children. Arch Otolaryngol Head Neck Surg 2004;130(2):171–5.
11. Walke M, Shankar L, Hawke M, et al. Maxillary sinus hypoplasia, embryology, and radiology. Arch Otolaryngol Head Neck Surg 2000;126:831–6.
12. Merck W. Pathogenic relationship between adenoid vegetations and maxillary sinusitis in children. HNO 1974;22(6):198–9.
13. Fukuda K, Matsune S, Ushikai M, et al. A study of the relationship between adenoid vegetation and rhinosinusitis. Am J Otolaryngol 1989;10(3):214–6.
14. Wang DY, Bernheim N, Kaufman L, et al. Assessment of adenoid size in children by fibreoptic examination. Clin Otolaryngol Allied Sci 1997;22(2):172–7.
15. Tuncer U, Aydogan B, Soylu L, et al. Chronic rhinosinusitis and adenoid hyper-trophy in children. Am J Otolaryngol 2004;25(1):5–10.
16. Bercin AS, Ural A, Kutluhan A, et al. Relationship between sinusitis and adenoid size in pediatric age group. Ann Otol Rhinol Laryngol 2007;116(7):550–3.
17. Rachelesfky GS, Goldberg M, Katz RM, et al. Sinus disease in children with respiratory allergy. J Allergy Clin Immunol 1978;61:310–4.
18. Furukawa CT. The role of allergy in sinusitis in children. J Allergy Clin Immunol 1992;90:515–7.
19. Tosca A, Riccio AM, Marseglia GL, et al. Nasal endoscopy in asthmatic children: assessment of rhinosinusitis and adenoiditis incidence, correlations with cytology and microbiology. Clin Exp Allergy 2001;31:609–15.
20. Leo G, Piacentini E, Consonni D, et al. Chronic rhinosinusitis and allergy. Pediatr Allergy Immunol 2007;18(S):19–21.

21. Di Domenicantonio R, De Savio M, Sammarro S, et al. Asthma and allergies in childhood in the city of Rome: the Italian contribution to the International Study on Allergies and Asthma in Childhood (ISAAC). Epidemiol Prev 2003;27:226–33.
22. Passalacqua G, Ciprandi G, Canonica GW. United airways disease: therapeutic implications. Thorax 2000;55:S26–7.
23. Baroody FM, Hughes CA, McDowell P, et al. Eosinophilia in chronic childhood sinusitis. Arch Otolaryngol Head Neck Surg 1995;121(12):1396–402.
24. Driscoll PV, Naclerio RM, Baroody FM. CD4+ lymphocytes are present in the sinus mucosa of children with chronic sinusitis. Arch Otolaryngol Head Neck Surg 1996;122(10):1071–6.
25. Chan KH, Abzug MJ, Coffinet L, et al. Chronic sinusitis in young children differs from adults: a histopathology study. J Pediatr 2004;144:206–12.
26. Barbero GJ. Gastroesophageal reflux and upper airway disease. Otolaryngol Clin North Am 1996;29:27–38.
27. Bothwell MR, Parsons DS, Talbot A, et al. Outcome of reflux therapy on pediatric chronic sinusitis. Otolaryngol Head Neck Surg 1999;21:255–61.
28. Vandenplas Y, Sacre-Smits L. Continuous 24-hour esophageal pH monitoring in 285 asymptomatic infants 0-15 months old. J Pediatr Gastroenterol Nutr 1987; 6(2):220–4.
29. Phipps CD, Wood WE, Gibson WS, et al. Gastroesophageal reflux contributing to chronic sinus disease in children. Arch Otolaryngol Head Neck Surg 2000;126: 831–6.
30. Babinski D, Trawinska-Bartnicka M. Rhinosinusitis in cystic fibrosis: not a simple story. Int J Pediatr Otorhinolaryngol 2008;72:619–24.
31. Lee D, Rosenfeld RM. Adenoid bacteriology and sinonasal symptoms in children. Otolaryngol Head Neck Surg 1997;116:301–7.
32. Shin KS, Jeong JH, et al. The role of adenoids in pediatric rhinosinusitis. Int J Pediatr Otorhinolaryngol 2008;72:1643–50.
33. Bernstein JM, Dryja D, Murphy TF. Molecular typing of paired bacterial isolates from the adenoid and lateral wall of the nose in children undergoing adenoidectomy: Implications in acute rhinosinusitis. Otolaryngol Head Neck Surg 2001;125: 593–7.
34. Coticchia J, Zuliani G, Coleman C, et al. Biofilm surface area in the pediatric nasopharynx: chronic rhinosinusitis vs. obstructive sleep apnea. Arch Otolaryngol Head Neck Surg 2007;133:110–4.
35. Briggs RD, Wright ST, Cordes S, et al. Smoking in chronic rhinosinusitis: a predictor of poor long-term outcome after endoscopic sinus surgery. Laryngoscope 2004;114(1):126–8.
36. Tamashiro E, Xiong G, Anselmo-Lima WT, et al. Cigarette exposure impairs respiratory epithelial ciliogenesis. Am J Rhinol Allergy 2009;23(2):117–22.
37. Chan KH, Winslow CP, Levin M, et al. Clinical practice guidelines for the management of chronic sinusitis in children. Otolaryngol Head Neck Surg 1999;120: 328–34.
38. Otten HW, Antvelink JP, Ruyter D, et al. Is antibiotic treatment of chronic sinusitis effective in children? Clin Otolaryngol 1994;19:215–7.
39. Otten FWA. Conservative treatment of chronic maxillary sinusitis in children. Acta Otorhinolaryngol Belg 1997;51:173–5.
40. Parsons DS. Chronic sinusitis: a medical or surgical disease? Otolaryngol Clin North Am 1996;29:1–9.
41. Rosenfeld RM. Pilot study of outcomes in pediatric rhinosinusitis. Arch Otolaryngol Head Neck Surg 1995;121:729–36.

42. Clement PAR, Bluestone CD, Gordts F, et al. Management of rhinosinusitis in children. Int J Pediatr Otorhinolaryngol 1999;49(S1):S95–100.
43. Huang WH, Fang SY. High prevalence of antibiotic resistance in isolates from the middle meatus of children and adults with acute rhinosinusitis. Am J Rhinol 2004; 18(6):387–91.
44. Keech DR, Ramadan H, Mathers P. Analysis of aerobic bacterial strains found in chronic rhinosinusitis using the polymerase chain reaction. Otolaryngol Head Neck Surg 2000;123(4):363–7.
45. Novembre E, Mori F, Pucci N, et al. Systemic treatment of rhinosinusitis in children. Pediatr Allergy Immunol 2007;18(Suppl):56–61.
46. Park CS, Park YS, Park YJ, et al. The inhibitory effects of macrolide antibiotics on bone remodeling in chronic rhinosinusitis. Otolaryngol Head Neck Surg 2007; 137(2):274–9.
47. Jaffe A, Francis J, Rosenthal M, et al. Long-term azithromycin may improve lung function in children with cystic fibrosis. Lancet 1998;351:420.
48. Suzuki H, Shimomura A, Ikeda K, et al. Inhibitory effect of macrolides on interleukin-8 secretion from cultured human nasal epithelial cells. Laryngoscope 1997;107:1661–6.
49. Bhattacharyya N. Antimicrobial therapy in chronic rhinosinusitis. Curr Allergy Asthma Rep 2009;9(3):221–6.
50. Adappa ND, Coticchia JM. Management of refractory chronic rhinosinusitis in children. Am J Otolaryngol 2006;27:384–9.
51. Stankiewicz JA, Musgrave BK, Scianna JM. Nasal amphotericin irrigation in chronic sinusitis. Curr Opin Otolaryngol Head Neck Surg 2008;16:44–6.
52. Ponikau JU, Sherris DA, Kern EB, et al. The diagnosis and incidence of allergic fungal sinusitis. Mayo Clin Proc 1999;74:877–84.
53. Ponikau JU, Sherris DA, Kita H, et al. Intranasal antifungal treatment in 51 patients with chronic rhinosinusitis. J Allergy Clin Immunol 2002;110:862–6.
54. Ponikau JU, Sherris DA, Weaver A, et al. Treatment of chronic rhinosinusitis with intranasal amphotericin B: a randomized, placebo-controlled, double-blind pilot trial. J Allergy Clin Immunol 2005;115:125–31.
55. Weschta M, Rimek D, Formanek M, et al. Topical antifungal treatment of chronic rhinosinusitis with nasal polyps: a randomized, double-blind clinical trial. J Allergy Clin Immunol 2004;114:1122–8.
56. Ebbens FA, Scadding GK, Badia L, et al. Amphotericin B nasal lavages: not a solution for patients with chronic rhinosinusitis. J Allergy Clin Immunol 2006;118:1149–56.
57. Weschta M, Rimek D, Formanek M, et al. Effect of nasal antifungal therapy on nasal cell activiation markers in chronic rhinosinusitis. Arch Otolaryngol Head Neck Surg 2006;132:743–7.
58. Tosca MA, Cosentino C, Pallestrini E, et al. Improvement of clinical and immunopathologic parameters in asthmatic children treated for concomitant chronic rhinosinusitis. Ann Allergy Asthma Immunol 2003;91(1):71–8.
59. Tosca MA, Cosentino C, Palletrini E, et al. Medical treatment reverses cytokine pattern in allergic and nonallergic chronic sinusitis in asthmatic children. Pediatr Allergy Immunol 2003;14:238–41.
60. Rachelefsky GS, Katz RM, Siegel SC. Chronic sinus disease with associated reactive airway disease. Pediatrics 1984;73(4):526–9.
61. Fiocchi A, Sarratud T, Bouygue GR, et al. Topical treatment of rhinosinusitis. Pediatr Allergy Immunol 2007;18(Suppl):62–7.
62. Dubin MG, Liu C, Lin SY, et al. American Rhinologic Society member survey on "maximal medical therapy" for chronic rhinosinusitis. Am J Rhinol 2007;21(4):483–8.

63. Schenkel EJ, Skoner DP, Bronsky EA. Absence of growth retardation in children with perennial allergic rhinitis after one year treatment with mometasone furoate aqueous nasal spray. Pediatrics 2000;105:e22.

64. Brannan MD, Herron JM, Affrime MB. Safety and tolerability of once-daily mometasone furoate aqueous nasal spray in children. Clin Ther 1997;19:1330–9.

65. Desrosiers MY, Kilty SJ. Treatment alternatives for chronic rhinosinusitis persisting after ESS: what to do when antibiotics, steroids and surgery fail. Rhinology 2008; 46(1):3–14.

66. Chiu AG, Palmer JN, Woodworth BA, et al. Baby shampoo nasal irrigations for the symptomatic post-functional sinus surgery patient. Am J Rhinol 2008;22(1): 34–7.

67. Ramadan HH. Adenoidectomy vs. endoscopic sinus surgery for the treatment of pediatric sinusitis. Arch Otolaryngol Head Neck Surg 1999;125:1208–11.

68. Takahashi H, Honjo I, Fujita A, et al. Effects of adenoidectomy on sinusitis. Acta Otorhinolaryngol Belg 1997;51:85–7.

69. Vanderberg SJ, Heatley DG. Efficacy of adenoidectomy in relieving symptoms of chronic sinusitis in children. Arch Otolaryngol Head Neck Surg 1997;123:675–8.

70. Ramadan HH. Surgical management of chronic sinusitis in children. Laryngoscope 2004;114:2103–9.

71. Buchman CA, Yellon RF, Bluestone CD. Alternative to endoscopic sinus surgery in the management of pediatric chronic rhinosinusitis refractory to oral antibiotic therapy. Otolaryngol Head Neck Surg 1999;120:219–24.

72. Don DM, Yellon RF, Casselbrant ML, et al. Efficacy of a stepwise protocol that includes intravenous antibiotic therapy for the management of chronic sinusitis in children and adolescents. Arch Otolaryngol Head Neck Surg 2001;127: 1093–8.

73. Ramadan HH, Cost JL. Outcome of adenoidectomy versus adenoidectomy with maxillary sinus wash for chronic rhinosinusitis in children. Laryngoscope 2008; 118:871–3.

74. Kaliner MA, Osguthorpe JD, Fireman P, et al. Sinusitis: bench to bedside – current findings, future directions. Otolaryngol Head Neck Surg 1997;116:301–7.

75. Lusk RP, Stankiewicz JA. Pediatric rhinosinusitis. Otolaryngol Head Neck Surg 1997;117:S53–7.

76. Bothwell MR, Piccirillo JF, Lusk RP, et al. Long-term outcome of facial growth after functional endoscopic sinus surgery. Otolaryngol Head Neck Surg 2002;126: 628–34.

77. Senior B, Wirtschafter A, Mai C, et al. Quantitative impact of pediatric sinus surgery on facial growth. Laryngoscope 2000;110:1866–70.

78. Kennedy DW, Zinreich SJ, Rosenbaum AE, et al. Functional endoscopic sinus surgery: theory and diagnostic evaluation. Arch Otolaryngol Head Neck Surg 1985;111:576–82.

79. Lusk RP, Muntz HR. Endoscopic sinus surgery in children with chronic sinusitis: a pilot study. Laryngoscope 1990;100:654–8.

80. Hebert RL, Bent JP. Meta-analysis of outcomes of pediatric functional endoscopic sinus surgery. Laryngoscope 1998;108:796–9.

81. Younis RT, Lazar RH. Criteria for success in pediatric functional endoscopic sinus surgery. Laryngoscope 1996;106:869–73.

82. Younis RT. The pros and cons of second-look sinonasal endoscopy after endoscopic sinus surgery in children. Arch Otolaryngol Head Neck Surg 2005; 131:267–9.

83. Parikh SR, Cuellar H, Sadoughi B, et al. Indications for image-guidance in pediatric sinonasal surgery. Int J Pediatr Otorhinolaryngol 2009;73:351–6.
84. Ramadan HH. Revision sinus surgery in children: surgical causes of failure. Laryngoscope 2009;199:1214–7.
85. Parsons DS, Greene BA. A treatment for primary ciliary dyskinesia: efficacy of functional endoscopic sinus surgery. Laryngoscope 1993;103:1269–72.
86. Ryan MW. Diseases associated with chronic rhinosinusitis: What is the significance? Curr Opin Otolaryngol Head Neck Surg 2008;16:231–6.
87. Cho DY, Hwang PH. Results of endoscopic maxillary mega-antrostomy in recalcitrant maxillary sinusitis. Am J Rhinol 2008;22:658–62.
88. Chee L, Graham SM, Carothers DG, et al. Immune dysfunction in refractory sinusitis in a tertiary care setting. Laryngoscope 2001;111:233–5.
89. Murphy C, Davidson TM, Jellison W, et al. Sinonasal disease and olfactory impairment in HIV disease: endoscopic sinus surgery and outcome measure. Laryngoscope 2000;110:1707–10.
90. Campbell JM, Graham M, Gray HC, et al. Allergic fungal sinusitis in children. Ann Allergy Asthma Immunol 2006;96:286–90.

When Surgery, Antibiotics, and Steroids Fail to Resolve Chronic Rhinosinusitis

Berrylin J. Ferguson, MD*, Bradley A. Otto, MD, Harshita Pant, BMBS, PhD

KEYWORDS

- Omalizumab • Zileuton • Immunodeficiency • Adenoiditis
- Aspirin • Desensitization • Montelukast • Odontogenic
- Sinusitis

Chronic rhinosinusitis (CRS) is a clinical syndrome encompassing a heterogeneous group of diseases characterized by sinonasal mucosal inflammation for at least 12 consecutive weeks.[1] Culture-directed antibiotic therapy and systemic and intranasal corticosteroid (INCS) therapy are considered the mainstay therapies for CRS. Consensus documents from the Rhinosinusitis Task Force and European Position Paper on Rhinosinusitis and Nasal Polyps codify diagnostic criteria and treatment strategies to guide and streamline CRS management.[1] This article discusses recalcitrant CRS after standard medical therapy and primary endoscopic sinus surgery (ESS). Optimal management is centered on a rational approach designed to identify and treat underlying etiologic and exacerbating factors, to maximize antiinflammatory therapy, and to ensure that confounding causes of sinus symptoms are addressed.

CONFOUNDING LOCAL AND REGIONAL FACTORS THAT MIMIC PURULENT CRS

Endoscopy and sinus computed tomography (CT) scan are essential to the diagnosis of CRS, and both techniques are useful in evaluating local and regional processes that mimic purulent CRS (**Box 1**). With endoscopy, the presence of a foreign body or tumor should be readily apparent.

Adenoiditis is less obvious although recognized as the primary source of nasal purulence in children. In adults, persistent mucopurulent postnasal drainage may be secondary to an infected Thornwaldt diverticulum or bursa. A Thornwaldt bursa represents the embryonic remnant of adhesion of the pharyngeal ectoderm to the cranial end of the notochord. If this becomes closed at the orifice, a cyst develops. Remnants

---

Division of Sinonasal Disorders and Allergy, Department of Otolaryngology, University of Pittsburgh School of Medicine, University of Pittsburgh Medical Center Mercy, 1400 Locust Street, Suite B11500, Pittsburgh, PA 15219, USA
* Corresponding author.
E-mail address: fergusonbj@upmc.edu (B.J. Ferguson).

Immunol Allergy Clin N Am 29 (2009) 719–732
doi:10.1016/j.iac.2009.07.009
0889-8561/09/$ – see front matter
immunology.theclinics.com

Box 1
Differential diagnosis of chronic rhinosinusitis in patients with mucopurulence

Sinonasal

    Rhinitis (acute, chronic)

    Foreign body

    Neoplasia

Locoregional

    Adenoiditis

    Thornwaldt cyst

    Dental abscess

    Neoplasia

---

that fail to close, and instead form a diverticulum, may be a source of repeated episodes of purulent postnasal drainage in the absence of sinus pathology. Treatment is endoscopic marsupialization or removal.

Underlying dental pathology should be considered in any patient with recalcitrant purulent CRS, particularly those with unilateral disease. Identification of dental disease not only helps with appropriate antibiotic selection but also facilitates improved long-term outcomes.[2,3] Sinus CT is helpful in assessing periodontal disease or periapical abscess as a cause of sinusitis and is more sensitive than plain dental films or a panorex.[4] A recent study showed that more than 80% of CT scans with maxillary sinus fluid levels greater than two-thirds the height of the sinus and with mucosal thickening had dental pathology compared with 10% incidence of dental pathology in normal maxillary sinuses.[4] Not all patients have specific dental symptoms or signs. However, once the diagnosis is established, appropriate treatment of the offending tooth by dental surgeons frequently obviates the need for sinus procedures. Directed endoscopic sinus surgery is reserved for situations in which persistent edema prevents maxillary sinus drainage.

LOCOREGIONAL AND SYSTEMIC FACTORS ASSOCIATED WITH PERSISTENT DISEASE

In persistent CRS (after medical therapy and primary ESS), locoregional and systemic factors known to be predictive of failed ESS include smoking, allergies,[5] and asthma and aspirin intolerance.[6,7] Additional factors that can play a role in actual or simulated persistent sinus symptoms include gastroesophageal reflux disease (GERD) and allergies.

Gastroesophageal Reflux Disease

GERD is associated with CRS in several studies; however, there is no direct evidence of causality.[8] In a prospective trial using pH probe monitoring, acid reflux into the nasopharynx was significantly greater in patients with refractory CRS after surgery than in patients in whom ESS successfully relieved symptoms. DelGaudio[9] suggested that there was an association between GERD and recalcitrant CRS. An alternative explanation for failure could be that CRS was not causing the patient's symptoms; rather the inadequately treated GERD caused the symptoms, as the sensation of post-nasal discharge can be simulated by pharyngeal and glottic irritation from GERD. Proton pump inhibitors can reduce the frequency of postnasal drainage symptoms in patients with extraesophageal manifestations of GERD.[10] An open-label study showed decreased sinonasal symptom scores in patients treated with omeprazole twice daily for 3 months.[11] No prospective, randomized controlled trials show the effectiveness of antireflux regimens in treating CRS.

Allergy

The association of allergic rhinitis (AR) and CRS is conflicting.[12,13] Patients with the most extensive disease on sinus CT are less likely to be allergic or to respond to allergy management than patients with lesser sinus disease. Houser and Keen[5] implicated AR as a predictive factor for decreased quality of life and poorer surgical outcomes in CRS. Although there is no evidence linking the pathogenesis of AR with CRS, the mucosal changes due to AR can alter mucociliary clearance, which can negatively affect CRS. In addition, AR symptoms such as drainage and nasal congestion mimic CRS symptoms. Management of concomitant AR is important in the comprehensive management of CRS; many symptoms are common to both conditions.

ALLERGY MANAGEMENT

The senior author (BJF) prefers to prescribe a treatment algorithm that includes progressive addition or replacement of various medications described in this section, including INCS, to arrive at a treatment regimen that is optimal for the individual. The cornerstone of this "rational patient experiment" is that the patient introduces 1 medication at a time for a sufficient duration to determine its efficacy in managing symptoms. The algorithm is provided to the patient in written form for reference until the next visit (**Table 1**). Immunotherapy is generally reserved for those with inadequate relief with environmental controls and medical therapy or for those with symptoms for at least 6 months of the year, so that the potential for cure is worth the time and small risks of immunotherapy. A detailed discussion of immunotherapy is beyond the scope of this article; however, it should be noted that immunotherapy is currently the only allergy treatment that offers a chance for a cure of AR symptoms.

Antihistamines

Histamine released from mast cells is responsible for most early phase symptoms of AR (sneezing, itching, and edema) by interaction with the H1 receptor. First-generation antihistamines (diphenhydramine, hydroxyzine, chlorpheniramine, and brompheniramine) can be sedating, can impair performance, and can exacerbate dryness, urinary retention, and narrow-angle glaucoma because of anticholinergic effects. Newer second-generation antihistamines are generally nonsedating, or have a lower sedating profile, and lack anticholinergic effects. Oral antihistamines are poor nasal decongestants; however, topical antihistamines are similar to INCS in terms of their symptom-relieving effect but with a more rapid onset of action. Side effects of topical antihistamines (azelastine HCl and olopatadine) include sedation (2%) and perverse taste. Concomitant usage with INCS may increase the control of symptoms.[14]

Decongestants

Decongestants are used for acute events and have little role in CRS. Common oral decongestants include pseudoephedrine and phenylephrine. Topical decongestants, including oxymetazoline and phenylephrine, also receive widespread use for nasal congestion because of the rapid onset of action; however, chronic use causes rebound congestion and tachyphylaxis.

Table 1
The rational patient experiment

Try Each Medicine in the Order Indicated	Medication	Dose	Number of Times a Day	Symptoms Which Should Improve and How Long it Should Take to Work	Check if Sample Given
	Nasal steroid spray Generic fluticasone propionate (Flonase) Triamcinolone (Nasacort) Mometasone furoate monohydrate (Nasonex) Budesonide (Rhinocort AQ) Fluticasone furoate (Veramyst) Ciclesonide (Omnaris) If any of the above are effective, let us know which ones on your formulary	1–2 puffs each nostril. Direct spray using right hand to spray left nose, and vice versa to maximize delivery laterally	1–2 times, use lowest dose that relieves symptoms	Nasal congestion, drainage, allergy symptoms—may take a week to work Slow to act	
	Antihistamine nasal spray Azelastine (Astelin) Azelastine (Astepro) Olopatadine (Patanase)	As above. Lean forward and do not sniff × 1 minute to minimize bad taste	2 times, take first dose before bedtime to see if it makes you sleepy	Nasal congestion, drainage, itch May work in less than half an hour Fast	
	Montelukast (Singulair)	10-mg pill	1 time	As above plus cough, fast	
	Antihistamines Loratadine (over the counter), Fexofenadine (Allegra) Levocetirizine (Xyzal), Cetirizine (Zyrtec)		1 time	Itch, sneeze Fast	

Medicine	Dose	Frequency	Notes
Guaifenesin (Mucinex)	600 mg	2 pills 2 times	Over the counter, less expensive generic on the Internet
Proton pump inhibitor			Take 0.5–1 h before a meal
Antibiotic			Eat yogurt, kefir, or take probiotics or acidophilus tablets (over the counter, health food store) while on an antibiotic to replenish good bacteria in your system
Saline nasal rinse Neil Med; Simply Saline (Blairex Laboratories, Inc., Columbus, Indiana), etc.			Use saline rinses before applying prescription nasal sprays
Queen Helene cocoa butter cream	Apply to front of nose	As needed	Available at Rite Aid, Wal-Mart, and on the Internet

Try each checked medicine one at a time.
If the medicine does not make you feel better in 3 to 4 days, then stop the medicine and try the next medicine listed.
If the medicine makes you feel partially better but not completely symptom free, then add the next medicine listed to the medicine that was partially helping you.
If the medicine relieves your symptoms, then continue it for at least several days or weeks. If you are feeling back to normal, then stop the medicine, but restart it if your symptoms start to return.

Anticholinergic Sprays

Ipratropium bromide, a topical anticholinergic nasal spray, blocks parasympathetic input to mucus glands and reduces rhinorrhea. Although decreased mucus production is desirable in some settings, it may lead to increased thickness of secretions and paradoxically worsen perceived postnasal drainage. It is formulated as a 0.03% solution for the treatment of AR rhinorrhea and a 0.06% solution for the treatment of rhinorrhea from the common cold.

Leukotriene Receptor Antagonists

Leukotrienes are produced about 1.5 hours into the allergic response, and their synthesis begins with oxidation of arachidonic acid from membrane phospholipids. Leukotriene effects include bronchoconstriction, increased vascular permeability, and leukocyte recruitment.

Montelukast blocks the cysteinyl-leukotriene receptor and is approved for asthma and seasonal and perennial AR. Montelukast added to INCS can improve symptom scores in CRS patients. As with all medications, some patients respond, others do not. The safety profile is excellent; however, in June 2009, the Food and Drug Administration (FDA) required that a warning of increased risk of neuropsychiatric events, including suicide and depression, be included in the label of all cysteinyl-leukotriene receptor antagonists. It is the authors' practice to give the patient a 1-week trial of therapy, and if no improvement in AR or CRS symptoms is noted, the patient is told not to fill the prescription.

Zileuton inhibits the 5-lipoxygenase enzyme and can inhibit leukotriene effects more potently than montelukast. In a randomized controlled study, a significant improvement in olfaction was noted in patients with CRS and concomitant aspirin sensitive asthma treated with zileuton.[15] Zileuton is only approved for asthma, and the dosage is zileuton CR 600 mg twice a day. Liver function (alanine transaminase [ALT] level) should be monitored monthly for 3 months. Up to 2% of patients on zileuton will experience an elevation in ALT, which normalizes on cessation of the medication.

Mast Cell Stabilizers

Mast cell stabilizers prevent histamine release from mast cells, most likely by calcium channel modulation. These medications do not affect the downstream effects of histamine, and therefore are only effective as prophylaxis. Cromolyn sodium nasal spray should be taken 4 times daily, which often compromises compliance. There are no serious side effects reported with this medication, and it can be used during pregnancy.

SYSTEMIC DISEASES AND ASSOCIATED MEDICAL CONDITIONS
Immune Deficiency

Immunodeficiency is estimated to occur in 8% to 20% of patients with persistent or recurrent acute sinusitis. Before effective antiretroviral therapy for human immunodeficiency virus (HIV), sinusitis was a common finding in the acquired immune deficiency syndrome. CRS associated with immunodeficiency may be responsive to antibiotic therapy but recurs when antibiotics are withdrawn.[16] The most common primary immunodeficiency in adults, the common variable immune deficiency (CVID), is reported to occur in up to 10% of patients with refractory CRS, whereas general immunoglobulin deficiencies are as high as 22% in the same population.[17,18] Because CVID is associated with additional risks, such as autoimmunity and malignancy, an accurate diagnosis has ramifications beyond CRS. CVID is treated with replacement immunoglobulin G; however, other identified immunodeficiencies may not be treatable. Identification is important because it alerts the physician and patient that the likelihood of an infection in this patient is greater and culture-directed antibiotics should be administered more promptly than in patients with normal immunity. IgA deficiency is less common in the CRS population than in the population at large.[19]

A general workup of immunity by the senior author (BJF) is displayed in **Box 2**. Costs of such a workup are less than the cost of a sinus CT scan. In addition, any patient suffering from recurrent acute infections should be offered a pneumococcal vaccine, which will theoretically immunize him or her to most, but not all, streptococcal pneumonia serotypes. Specific polysaccharide antibody deficiency syndrome is diagnosed by deficient responses to pneumococcal vaccine comparing the levels before 6 weeks after vaccination, in the context of normal systemic immunoglobulin levels.[20]

Asthma and Sensitivity to Aspirin and Analgesics

The triad of sinusitis, bronchial asthma, and aspirin intolerance is known as Widal syndrome, Samter triad, and aspirin exacerbated respiratory disease (AERD). Patients with CRS with nasal polyps (NPs) are more likely to have aspirin hypersensitivity or asthma than the general population. NPs are reported in up to 70% of aspirin-intolerant patients with asthma. Aspirin or analgesic intolerance is not always associated with the full clinical picture of NPs and asthma but may be restricted to just the upper airway. In sensitive individuals, even a very small single dose of aspirin or other cyclooxygenase-1 (COX-1) inhibitor can cause rhinorrhea, bronchospasm, and shock. This mechanism is not caused by an IgE-mediated allergy; rather the reaction occurs because these individuals produce increased amounts of leukotrienes. Prostaglandin E2 (PGE2), produced by the cyclooxygenase pathway, is an inhibitor of 5-lipoxygenase and leukotriene production. A COX-1 inhibitor, such as aspirin, inhibits production of PGE2, causing a release of inhibition of the 5-lipoxygenase enzyme and an increase in leukotriene production. The gold standard for the diagnosis of AERD is an oral provocation test under close supervision. AERD patients may tolerate COX-2 inhibitors, and occasionally patients report improvement in symptoms on a COX-2 inhibitor, although the mechanism is unknown.[21]

Aspirin desensitization may be beneficial and must be performed under supervised conditions. Various aspirin doses (100–1300 mg) and routes of administration (oral, intranasal) are reported. Once desensitized, the patient must take aspirin daily. Failure to take aspirin for several days renders the patient hypersensitive to its effects once more. Up to 30% of patients cannot tolerate the side effects from daily aspirin therapy. Even though other COX-1 inhibitors such as ibuprofen can trigger bronchospasm in these individuals, to date, it has not been possible to desensitize a patient with any

---

Box 2
Immunodeficiency evaluation

Complete blood count with differential

Quantitative immunoglobulins: IgA, IgE, IgG, IgM

Immunoglobulin subclasses: secretory IgA, IgG1, IgG2, IgG3, IgG4

T-cell subpopulations: CD4, CD8

Pneumococcal antibody titers: before and 6 weeks after pneumococcal vaccination

agent except aspirin. Desensitization can improve asthma control and prevent continued growth of NPs, but it does not usually cause NP regression.[22]

Vasculitides and Granulomatous Disorders

Wegener's granulomatosis (WG) is a rare granulomatous vasculitic disorder, occurring in approximately 3 per 100,000 people, affecting primarily whites (97%) aged between 50 and 60 years.[23–25] Sinonasal manifestations occur in up to 89% of patients.[23] Common symptoms include nasal obstruction, rhinorrhea (frequently bloody), epiphora, and crusting. Patients may present with recalcitrant CRS, septal perforation, mucocele, orbital pseudotumor, or saddle-nose deformity. In patients with clinical features consistent with WG, positive cytoplasmic antineutrophil cytoplasmic antibodies and an elevated erythrocyte sedimentation rate suggest the diagnosis. However, definitive diagnosis depends on histopathologic analysis of affected mucosa.[26] Treatment of WG should be given in consultation with a rheumatologist.

Churg-Strauss syndrome (CSS) is characterized by multisystem granulomatous eosinophilic tissue infiltration. Nasal involvement can occur in up to 75% of patients. Clinical presentation is similar to WG, with the exception of a more profound and systemic neuropathy. Diagnosis is based on clinical findings, positive perinuclear antineutrophil cytoplasmic antibodies, and biopsy.

Sarcoidosis, an inflammatory multisystem disorder of uncertain etiology, is characterized by noncaseating granulomas. Although the lower respiratory tract is frequently involved, the sinonasal cavity is affected in only 0.7% to 6% of cases.[27] Common examination findings include mucosal hypertrophy, purple mucosa with nodules (granulomas), and lupus pernio.[26,27] Diagnosis is based on clinical findings, chest radiography, elevated angiotensin-converting enzyme levels, and findings of mucosal biopsy from affected mucosa.[26] Treatment of CSS and sarcoidosis often requires oral steroids and immunosuppressants, and surgery is reserved for extreme or complicated cases.

OPTIMIZING MEDICAL THERAPY FOR PERSISTENT CRS

An assessment of compliance and an evaluation of treatments that have worked or have not worked for the patient should be undertaken at every visit to facilitate stepwise introduction and testing of efficacy of various therapeutic interventions. In addition to allergy medications, including leukotriene modulators that are discussed in the allergy section, this section completes the discussion of available medical therapies, beyond steroids and antibiotics (**Box 3**).

Antifungals

In double-blind randomized controlled trials, the topical antifungal amphotericin is no more effective in reducing CT scan scores than saline (level 1 evidence).[28,29] In another double-blind, placebo-controlled study, oral terbinafine failed to improve symptoms or radiographic appearance of CRS.[30] In a retrospective review of 23 patients from Australia with refractory allergic fungal sinusitis (AFS) and nonallergic fungal sinusitis, use of the antifungal oral agent itraconazole 100 mg twice daily for 6 months led to improvement of refractory disease in 19 patients, with 11 patients disease-free at 6 months.[31]

Three patients had to stop the itraconazole because of elevated liver enzymes. Earlier randomized controlled studies on topical antifungals did not specifically enroll patients with evidence of eosinophilic fungal disease, which could explain the differences in findings in these studies. A randomized controlled study of patients with

---

Box 3
Medical treatment options for chronic rhinosinusitis: beyond steroids, antibiotics, and surgery

Treatment strategies

Antifungals

   Topical and systemic

Allergy management

   Antihistamines

      Topical sprays, oral

   Allergen avoidance

      Fix water leaks, avoid dust mites, use BreathePure (Breathepure Healthcare, LLC, Santa Barbara, California) nasal filters

   Immunotherapy

      Subcutaneous, sublingual

Food allergy

   Elimination challenge diet

Topical saline irrigation

   Hypotonic, hypertonic, isotonic

Mucus modifiers

   Guaifenesin

   Anticholinergics

Leukotriene modulators

   Leukotriene receptor antagonist (montelukast)

   5-Lipoxygenase inhibitor (zileuton)

Decongestants

   Topical

   Systemic

Diet modification

   Omega 3, vitamins, probiotics

Lifestyle modification

   Stop smoking, get adequate sleep, exercise regularly, avoid pollution

---

eosinophilic fungal disease is required to assess the efficacy of antifungal therapies in this subset of CRS patients.

Mucolytics

Mucolytics, including guaifenesin or acetylcysteine, decrease the viscosity of secretions in the upper airway, theoretically improving mucociliary transport. Guaifenesin has been approved for use by the FDA since 1952 and is a common component of over-the-counter cough and cold formulations. In a randomized placebo-controlled study in HIV-positive patients before effective antiretrovirals were available, guaifenesin at a dose of 1200 mg twice daily led to reduced congestion and postnasal drainage.[32] Because of the limited data related to CRS management, recommendations for or against mucolytic use cannot be clearly argued. However, with an excellent safety profile, use of mucolytics should not be discouraged in patients who perceive a benefit.

Topical Nasal Saline

Nasal saline is widely used in the treatment of CRS and is applied by various methods, including spray, nebulization, and irrigation. Nasal saline irrigations improve symptom scores and improve symptom control in CRS with persistent disease. Nasal saline irrigation can be used to deliver baby shampoo, sodium hypochlorite, xylitol, Dead Sea salt, and povidone-iodine (Betadine). None of these additions have been studied with a randomized controlled trial. In unoperated sinuses, the effect of saline irrigations is limited to the nasal cavity.

In cystic fibrosis (CF), hypertonic nasal saline may be more effective than isotonic saline. This is inferred from a double-blind randomized controlled study that showed hypertonic saline to be more effective than isotonic saline in pulmonary nebulization in patients with CF.[33] Up to 8% of CRS patients are heterozygotes for CF.[34] Potentially, CRS CF carriers may also benefit from hypertonic saline irrigations; other CRS patients would benefit from isotonic irrigations.

Anti-IgE

Omalizumab (Xolair) is a monoclonal antibody that selectively binds to human IgE and is currently approved for use in patients older than 12 years with moderate to severe persistent asthma with a positive skin test or in vitro reactivity to perennial aeroallergens and whose symptoms are inadequately controlled with inhaled corticosteroids. Other inflammatory conditions such as AR and CRS with NP have been reported to improve with omalizumab. Omalizumab has been reported to resolve allergic bronchopulmonary aspergillosis. The senior author (BJF) treated a patient with AFS who improved dramatically after starting omalizumab treatment. However, anti-IgE therapy is costly ($10,000–12,000 per year), somewhat inconvenient (requiring a shot once or twice a month), and carries potential risk (rare anaphylaxis has been reported), and a possible increased risk of cardiovascular and cerebrovascular adverse events.

Mepolizumab is an anti–interleukin-5 monoclonal antibody that binds to interleukin-5, the cytokine most potent in stimulating eosinophil production, activation, and maturation. Treatment with mepolizumab causes a sustained reduction in the number of circulating eosinophils because of its long terminal half-life.[35] Mepolizumab currently has an orphan drug status, and its use remains investigational in the treatment of hypereosinophilic syndrome. Its role in the treatment of AR and CRS has yet to be determined.

Food Allergy

Food allergy by prick testing is present in more than 70% of CRS patients with NP compared with only 34% of controls. The incidence of inhalant allergy by prick testing in patients with NP is only 35%.[36] Making this diagnosis is challenging, often because of an inability to clearly define the inciting foods and because skin prick tests and in vitro tests can miss this diagnosis, as many food hypersensitivities may not be IgE-mediated. The gold standard for diagnosis of food allergy is a double-blind, placebo-controlled, oral challenge; however, this is often impractical. Patients can perform similar elimination challenge procedures at home. Although not blinded or controlled, this allows for a convenient inexpensive self-diagnosis. Most common "masked" food allergens in adults in the United States are those foods commonly eaten and include wheat, dairy, soy, corn, and, occasionally, eggs. To perform an elimination food challenge, the targeted food is eliminated from the diet for 5 to 7 days and then reintroduced into the diet during this hyperresponsive period of 5 to 10 days following elimination. If the food causes symptoms, then the patient will generally be aware of either nasal or nonnasal symptoms (fatigue, bloating, and abdominal cramping) within 15 minutes to 6 hours after the food challenge. Patients are advised to test for the 5 foods listed in succession. Those who note symptoms on reintroduction of the food are instructed to eliminate the food from their diet for approximately 3 months, after which time the food may be reintroduced into their diet, although the food should not be eaten on a daily basis.[37]

Lifestyle and Dietary Modifications

These factors are addressed to promote a healthier lifestyle that influences sinonasal health. Patients are encouraged to maintain adequate hydration with noncaffeinated drinks for optimal mucus quality. A study in patients with CF showed that dehydration was associated with increased biofilms, ineffective defense,[38] and decreased mucociliary clearance.[39] Other advice includes adequate exercise, cessation of smoking, and use of nasal air filters or masks to reduce exposure to inhaled allergens and pollution.

ALTERNATIVE THERAPIES

Alternatives therapies include acupuncture and several herbal remedies. There is little objective evidence of efficacy for these measures. A study on acupuncture showed no significant difference in health-related quality of life compared with conventional medical therapy, which consisted of 2 to 4 weeks of antibiotics, corticosteroids, 0.9% sodium chloride solution, and local decongestants.[40] The conventional treatment group had better symptom scores and physical scores than the acupuncture group.

Phototherapy using a combination of ultraviolet (UV) A and UV B and laser therapy can reduce mucosal inflammation by inducing apoptosis and functional alteration of lymphocytes, antigen-presenting cells and eosinophils, and by altering cytokine levels and other chemical mediators, including histamine. Phototherapy has been used to treat AR, and its use may extend to a select group of patients with CRS.[41] Preliminary studies show no adverse effect on the regenerative capacity of nasal epithelium.[42] The other immune modulatory and suppressive agents that have potential to either provide immunostimulation and protection or to reduce mucosal inflammation include microbial and T-cell vaccines, bacterial-derived stimulants (ribomunyl), and T-cell suppressants (pimecrolimus).

SUMMARY

Management of CRS can be complex, and definitive evidence-based protocols cannot be currently defined because of disease heterogeneity, incomplete understanding of refractory cases, and differences in individual responses to various interventions. An accurate diagnosis of CRS and treatment of associated conditions facilitates effective management. Included in the differential for purulent CRS mimics are adenoiditis, Thornwaldt cyst, and dental infection. Control of AR and GERD can provide symptom relief, if not necessarily improve sinusitis. Immunodeficiency, systemic granulomatous diseases, and vasculitides are systemic disorders that may predispose patients to recalcitrant CRS. Successful management is generally dependent on resolution or optimization of the underlying systemic disorder. Finally, in refractory patients, antifungals (in patients with positive fungal cultures and eosinophilic mucin), leukotriene modulators (montelukast /zileuton), aspirin desensitization (if aspirin-sensitive), and omalizumab (anti-IgE, for those with elevated IgE) may be beneficial. To determine empirically if the intervention is helpful, patients should introduce only 1 therapeutic variable at a time and monitor symptom response.

REFERENCES

1. Fokkens W, Lund V, Mullol J. European position paper on rhinosinusitis and nasal polyps 2007. Rhinol Suppl 2007;20:1–136.
2. Brook I. Microbiology of acute sinusitis of odontogenic origin presenting with periorbital cellulitis in children. Ann Otol Rhinol Laryngol 2007;116:386–8.
3. Legert KG, Zimmerman M, Stierna P. Sinusitis of odontogenic origin: pathophysiological implications of early treatment. Acta Otolaryngol 2004;124:655–63.
4. Bomeli SR, Branstetter BFt, Ferguson BJ. Frequency of a dental source for acute maxillary sinusitis. Laryngoscope 2009;119:580–4.
5. Houser SM, Keen KJ. The role of allergy and smoking in chronic rhinosinusitis and polyposis. Laryngoscope 2008;118:1521–7.
6. Wynn R, Har-El G. Recurrence rates after endoscopic sinus surgery for massive sinus polyposis. Laryngoscope 2004;114:811–3.
7. Robinson JL, Gries S, James KE, et al. Impact of aspirin intolerance on outcomes of sinus surgery. Laryngoscope 2007;117:825–30.
8. Passali D, Caruso G, Passali FM. ENT manifestations of gastroesophageal reflux. Curr Allergy Asthma Rep 2008;8:240–4.
9. DelGaudio JM. Direct nasopharyngeal reflux of gastric acid is a contributing factor in refractory chronic rhinosinusitis. Laryngoscope 2005;115:946–57.
10. Pawar S, Lim HJ, Gill M, et al. Treatment of postnasal drip with proton pump inhibitors: a prospective, randomized, placebo-controlled study. Am J Rhinol 2007;21:695–701.
11. DiBaise JK, Brand RE, Quigley EM. Endoluminal delivery of radiofrequency energy to the gastroesophageal junction in uncomplicated GERD: efficacy and potential mechanism of action. Am J Gastroenterol 2002;97:833–42.
12. Pearlman AN, Chandra RK, Chang D, et al. Relationships between severity of chronic rhinosinusitis and nasal polyposis, asthma, and atopy. Am J Rhinol Allergy 2009;23:145–8.
13. Emanuel IA, Shah SB. Chronic rhinosinusitis: allergy and sinus computed tomography relationships. Otolaryngol Head Neck Surg 2000;123:687–91.
14. Ratner PH, Hampel F, Van Bavel J, et al. Combination therapy with azelastine hydrochloride nasal spray and fluticasone propionate nasal spray in the treatment of patients with seasonal allergic rhinitis. Ann Allergy Asthma Immunol 2008;100:74–81.
15. Dahlen B, Nizankowska E, Szczeklik A, et al. Benefits from adding the 5-lipoxygenase inhibitor zileuton to conventional therapy in aspirin-intolerant asthmatics. Am J Respir Crit Care Med 1998;157:1187–94.
16. Kainulainen L, Suonpaa J, Nikoskelainen J, et al. Bacteria and viruses in maxillary sinuses of patients with primary hypogammaglobulinemia. Arch Otolaryngol Head Neck Surg 2007;133:597–602.
17. Chee L, Graham SM, Carothers DG, et al. Immune dysfunction in refractory sinusitis in a tertiary care setting. Laryngoscope 2001;111:233–5.
18. Vanlerberghe L, Joniau S, Jorissen M. The prevalence of humoral immunodeficiency in refractory rhinosinusitis: a retrospective analysis. B-ENT 2006;2:161–6.

19. Pant H, Kette FE, Smith WB, et al. Eosinophilic mucus chronic rhinosinusitis: clinical subgroups or a homogeneous pathogenic entity? Laryngoscope 2006; 116:1241–7.

20. Cheng YK, Decker PA, O'Byrne MM, et al. Clinical and laboratory characteristics of 75 patients with specific polysaccharide antibody deficiency syndrome. Ann Allergy Asthma Immunol 2006;97:306–11.

21. Block SH. Chronic sinusitis with rofecoxib. J Allergy Clin Immunol 2002;109: 373–4.

22. Stevenson DD, Hankammer MA, Mathison DA, et al. Aspirin desensitization treatment of aspirin-sensitive patients with rhinosinusitis-asthma: long-term outcomes. J Allergy Clin Immunol 1996;98:751–8.

23. Cannady SB, Batra PS, Koening C, et al. Sinonasal Wegener granulomatosis: a single-institution experience with 120 cases. Laryngoscope 2009;119: 757–61.

24. Fauci AS, Haynes BF, Katz P, et al. Wegener's granulomatosis: prospective clinical and therapeutic experience with 85 patients for 21 years. Ann Intern Med 1983;98:76–85.

25. McDonald TJ, DeRemee RA. Head and neck involvement in Wegener's granulomatosis (WG). Adv Exp Med Biol 1993;336:309–13.

26. Wytske J, Fokkens BR, Georgalas C. Pathophysiology of inflammation in the surgically failed sinus cavity. In: Stilianos E, Kountakis JBJ, Gosepath Jan, editors. Pathophysiology of inflammation in the surgically failed sinus cavity. Berlin, Heidelberg: Springer; 2008.

27. Aubart FC, Ouayoun M, Brauner M, et al. Sinonasal involvement in sarcoidosis: a case-control study of 20 patients. Medicine (Baltimore) 2006;85:365–71.

28. Weschta M, Rimek D, Formanek M, et al. Topical antifungal treatment of chronic rhinosinusitis with nasal polyps: a randomized, double-blind clinical trial. J Allergy Clin Immunol 2004;113:1122–8.

29. Ebbens FA, Scadding GK, Badia L, et al. Amphotericin B nasal lavages: not a solution for patients with chronic rhinosinusitis. J Allergy Clin Immunol 2006; 118:1149–56.

30. Kennedy DW, Kuhn FA, Hamilos DL, et al. Treatment of chronic rhinosinusitis with high-dose oral terbinafine: a double blind, placebo-controlled study. Laryngoscope 2005;115(10):1793–9.

31. Seiberling K, Wormald PJ. The role of itraconazole in recalcitrant fungal sinusitis. Am J Rhinol Allergy 2009;23:303–6.

32. Wawrose SF, Tami TA, Amoils CP. The role of guaifenesin in the treatment of sinonasal disease in patients infected with the human immunodeficiency virus (HIV). Laryngoscope 1992;102:1225–8.

33. Donaldson SH, Bennett WD, Zeman KL, et al. Mucus clearance and lung function in cystic fibrosis with hypertonic saline. N Engl J Med 2006;354:241–50.

34. Wang X, Moylan B, Leopold DA, et al. Mutation in the gene responsible for cystic fibrosis and predisposition to chronic rhinosinusitis in the general population. JAMA 2000;284:1814–9.

35. Mepolizumab: 240563, anti-IL-5 monoclonal antibody (abstract) GlaxoSmith Kline, Drugs in R&D 2008;9:125–30.

36. Collins MM, Loughran S, Davidson P, et al. Nasal polyposis: prevalence of positive food and inhalant skin tests. Otolaryngol Head Neck Surg 2006;135: 680–3.

37. Ozdemir O, Mete E, Catal F, et al. Food intolerances and eosinophilic esophagitis in childhood. Dig Dis Sci 2009;54:8–14.

38. Matsui H, Wagner VE, Hill DB, et al. A physical linkage between cystic fibrosis airway surface dehydration and *Pseudomonas aeruginosa* biofilms. Proc Natl Acad Sci U S A 2006;103:18131–6.

39. Kondo CS, Macchionne M, Nakagawa NK, et al. Effects of intravenous furosemide on mucociliary transport and rheological properties of patients under mechanical ventilation. Crit Care 2002;6:81–7.

40. Stavem K, Rossberg E, Larsson PG. Health-related quality of life in a trial of acupuncture, sham acupuncture, and conventional treatment for chronic sinusitis. BMC Res Notes 2008;1:37.

41. Kemeny L, Koreck A. Ultraviolet light phototherapy for allergic rhinitis. J Photochem Photobiol B, Biol 2007;87:58–65.

42. Koreck A, Szechenyi A, Morocz M, et al. Effects of intranasal phototherapy on nasal mucosa in patients with allergic rhinitis. J Photochem Photobiol B, Biol 2007;89:163–9.

Rhinosinusitis and the Lower Airways

Peter W. Hellings, MD, PhD*, Greet Hens, MD, PhD

KEYWORDS

- Rhinitis • Sinusitis • Asthma
- Chronic obstructive pulmonary disease • United airways

Due to its strategic position at the entry of the airway, the nose plays a crucial role in airway homeostasis.[1] By warming up, humidifying, and filtering incoming air, the nose is essential in the protection and homeostasis of lower airways. The nose and bronchi are anatomically connected, are lined with a pseudostratified respiratory epithelium, and equipped with an array of innate and acquired immune defense mechanisms. It is not hard to imagine that nasal conditions causing nasal obstruction, stasis of nasal secretions, or infectious disease of the sinonasal mucosa may become a trigger for lower airway pathology in susceptible individuals.[2] Common cold, acute rhinosinusitis, and chronic rhinosinusitis (CRS) are associated with nasal congestion or secretions in the sinonasal cavities impairing the protective function of the nose on the lower airways. In chronic sinus disease with nasal polyps (NP),[3] total blockage of the nasal passages may occur, hence bypassing the nasal effects on inspired air. It has become evident that the nasobronchial interaction is not limited to bronchial effects of impaired nasal breathing. Besides direct anatomic pathways, the nose and bronchi seem to communicate via indirect mechanisms. In contrast to ill-defined nasobronchial reflex mechanisms, rhinosinusitis is associated with a well-known systemic inflammation contributing to the interaction between nose and bronchi. The inflammation seen in CRS with or without NP shows systemic signs of inflammation such as elevated levels of interleukin (IL)-5 in the blood and increased bone marrow eosinopoiesis.[4] This article aims at providing a comprehensive overview of the current knowledge of nasobronchial communication in acute rhinosinusitis and CRS, including consequences for treatment.

INFECTIOUS RHINITIS AND LOWER AIRWAY DISEASE
Prevalence

It is obvious that common colds account for approximately 50% of all illnesses and are even more frequent in young infants.[5] Besides inducing nasal obstruction, rhinorrhea,

Department of Otorhinolaryngology, Head and Neck Surgery, University Hospitals Leuven, Catholic University of Leuven, Kapucijnenvoer 33, 3000 Leuven, Belgium
* Corresponding author.
E-mail address: peter.hellings@uzleuven.be (P.W. Hellings).

Immunol Allergy Clin N Am 29 (2009) 733–740
doi:10.1016/j.iac.2009.08.001   immunology.theclinics.com
0889-8561/09/$ – see front matter © 2009 Elsevier Inc. All rights reserved.

and sneezing, upper respiratory tract infections also cause exacerbations of preexisting lower airways diseases such as asthma or chronic obstructive pulmonary disease (COPD). The majority of asthma exacerbations are precipitated by respiratory virus infections in all age groups. When sensitive methods such as reverse transcription-polymerase chain reaction are used, viruses are found in 80% of wheezing episodes in school-aged children and in almost 50% of asthma exacerbations in adults. Rhinovirus (RV) is the most frequently detected pathogen.[6] The causal relationship between RV infection and asthma exacerbations has been proven by experimental infection models. After nebulization of an RV-16 suspension, asthma patients develop rhinitis symptoms together with worsening of their asthma state.[7] Moreover, a decrease in forced expiratory volume in 1 second (FEV1), increased airway hyperresponsiveness, and augmented eosinophilic bronchial inflammation are found following experimental RV infection.[7] Even in nonasthmatic patients with atopic rhinitis, RV inoculation increases airway hyperreactivity and induces a drop in FEV1.[8] Besides causing the majority of wheezing episodes in asthmatic patients, common colds are also associated with more than 40% of COPD exacerbations, with RV being the most common viral pathogen.[9]

Pathophysiology

The mechanisms of virus-induced exacerbations of asthma and COPD remain incompletely understood. A first question is whether RVs reach and replicate in the lower airways, causing lower airways symptoms by direct infection, or if indirect mechanisms are responsible for exacerbations of lower airways diseases. Recent evidence supports the first hypothesis. The presence of RV in bronchial biopsy specimens after experimental upper respiratory RV infection in human volunteers was confirmed by in situ hybridization and immunohistochemistry.[10,11] By using the latter methods, the investigators avoid contamination from the upper airways, which could not be excluded in studies where RV was detected in bronchoalveolar lavage or sputum. However, the importance of bronchial penetration and replication of RV during natural infection is still uncertain. Ninety percent of RVs infect airway epithelial cells via binding to the receptor ICAM-1, followed by intracellular penetration and replication. RVs upregulate the expression of ICAM-1 via nuclear factor (NF)-κB–dependent mechanisms, thereby enhancing their own infectivity and promoting inflammatory cell infiltration. In bronchial epithelial cell cultures, RV infection induces a variety of proinflammatory cytokines and chemokines such as IL-6, IL-8, IL-16, and RANTES, which may lead to the chemotaxis and activation of neutrophils, lymphocytes, monocytes, and eosinophils, thereby enhancing lower airway inflammation.[10] Besides a direct effect of RV on bronchial epithelial cells, indirect mechanisms could play a role in increasing lower airway inflammation during a common cold. Following experimental RV-16 infection in allergic individuals, granulocyte colony-stimulating macrophage (G-CSF) levels increase not only in nasal secretions but also in the circulation. G-CSF levels in serum correlate with the blood neutrophilia, suggesting that G-CSF acts on the bone marrow to increase the neutrophilia in blood.[12] Besides the proinflammatory effect of RV on airway epithelium, host factors also play an important role in the development of acute exacerbations. Several risk factors for experiencing more severe viral exacerbations of lower airway disease have been described, including age (being an infant or an elderly), smoking, and having low neutralizing antibody titers to RV.[12] Moreover, atopic asthmatic individuals are more prone to virus-induced wheezing, possibly via less interferon (IFN)-γ production in response to RV, which reflects a defective Th1 immune response. However, Avila and colleagues[13] showed a delayed onset of cold symptoms and a shortening of their duration when inoculation with RV was preceded by allergen challenge in subjects with allergic rhinitis. In this experimental setting, allergic inflammation may be protective for RV infection, probably depending on the timing and intensity of antigen exposure.

Treatment

Although acute viral exacerbations account for a large part of the burden associated with asthma and COPD, currently available treatments are unsatisfactory. Upper airway symptoms are not life-threatening but self-limiting. Therefore, treatment of upper airway symptoms is symptomatic, including nasal decongestants, rinsing of the nasal cavity, and oral analgesics if necessary.[3] To treat viral-induced asthma and COPD exacerbations, one can target either the virus itself or the host immune response. No RV vaccination exists because of the wide variety of serotypes of human RV. A range of antiviral agents has been tested in preclinical or clinical trials without consistent effects on asthma. Another therapeutic strategy is to prevent the inflammatory reaction caused by RV infection. Glucocorticosteroids are the cornerstone of current asthma and COPD maintenance therapy. However, they disappoint in the treatment of acute exacerbations. In persistent asthma, daily administration of inhaled corticosteroids has only a limited effect in reducing the number of wheezing episodes, both in adults and children. In exacerbations of COPD, corticosteroids have no major therapeutic efficacy as they reduce the absolute treatment failure rate by only 10%, increase the FEV1 by only 100 mL, and shorten the hospital stay by 1 to 2 days. Inhibiting the NF-κB signaling may also represent an interesting therapeutic option, because NF-κB is involved in both the virus-induced upregulation of ICAM-1 as well as in the transcriptional activation of a large number of the proinflammatory mediators involved in RV infection.[14] NF-κB inhibitors are, however, in an experimental stage of development, and it remains to be determined whether the anti-inflammatory properties of these agents will not be counterbalanced by the simultaneous inhibition of protective, antiviral mediators such as IFN.

RHINOSINUSITIS WITHOUT NASAL POLYPS AND ASTHMA
Prevalence

Bronchial asthma is considered a comorbidity of CRS.[3] In some centers, around 50% of patients with CRS have clinical asthma.[1] Of note, most patients with CRS who do not report to have asthma show bronchial hyperreactivity when given a metacholine challenge test.[15] In this way, Ponikau and colleagues[15] concluded that 91% of patients with CRS had either asthma or increased bronchial hyperreactivity. Others report that 60% of patients with CRS have lower airway involvement, assessed by history, pulmonary function, and histamine provocation tests.[3] Alternatively, sinonasal symptoms are frequently reported in asthmatic patients, ranging up to 80% in some studies. Radiologic imaging of the sinuses has demonstrated mucosal thickening of the sinus mucosa in up to 84% of patients with severe asthma. However, these epidemiologic and radiologic data should be interpreted with caution as they may reflect a large reference bias.[3]

Pathophysiology

CRS is currently thought to have a multifactorial etiology in which host factors like anatomic, local defense, and immunologic factors act in synergy with microbial and environmental factors.[3] Histopathologic features of CRS and asthma largely overlap.[3] Heterogeneous eosinophilic inflammation and features of airway remodeling such as epithelial shedding and basement membrane thickening are found in the mucosa of

CRS and asthma. Cytokine patterns in sinus tissue of CRS highly resemble those of bronchial tissue in asthma, explaining the presence of eosinophils in both conditions. Therefore, eosinophil degranulation proteins may cause damage to the surrounding structures and induce symptoms at their location in the airway. Finally, lavages from CRS patients show that eosinophils were the dominant cell type in both nasal and bronchoalveolar lavage in the subgroup of patients with CRS with asthma.[16] Besides the similarities in pathophysiology, sinusitis has been etiologically linked to bronchial asthma, and vice versa. As is the case in allergic airway inflammation, sinusitis and asthma can affect each other via the systemic route, involving IL-5 and the bone marrow. In both CRS and allergic asthma, similar proinflammatory markers are found in the blood. Nasal application of *Staphylococcus aureus* enterotoxin B has recently been shown to aggravate the allergen-induced bronchial eosinophilia in a mouse model.[17] Here, mucosal contact with enterotoxin B induced the systemic release of IL-4, IL-5, and IL-13, leading to aggravation of experimental asthma. However, the interaction between rhinosinusitis and asthma in not always clinically present, nor is there a consistent correlation between computed tomography scan abnormalities, sputum eosinophilia, and pulmonary function.[3]

Effects of Treatment of Chronic Rhinosinusitis on Bronchial Disease

Endoscopic sinus surgery (ESS) for CRS is most often successful for sinonasal symptoms, but may also improve bronchial symptoms and reduce medication use for bronchial asthma.[1] After a mean follow-up period of 6.5 years, 90% of asthmatic patients reported that their asthma was better than it had been before the ESS, with a reduction of the number of asthma attacks and medication use for asthma.[18] Also in children with sinusitis and asthma, sinus surgery improves the clinical course of asthma, reflected by a reduced number of asthma hospitalizations and schooldays missed.[19] Lung function in asthma patients with CRS was reported to benefit from ESS by some investigators, but this was denied by others.[1] Of note, not all studies show beneficial effects of ESS on asthma. The reason for the inconsistency in study results between studies relates to the heterogeneity and small number of patients included in these studies, and difference in outcome parameters studied. Of note, the presence of lower airway disease may have a negative impact on the outcome after ESS. Outcomes after ESS were significantly worse in the asthma compared with the non-asthma group.[1] Poor outcomes after ESS have also been reported in patients with aspirin-intolerant asthma.[19,20] On the other hand, other investigators report that asthma does not represent a predictor of poor symptomatic outcome after primary or revision ESS. In a series of 120 patients undergoing ESS, Kennedy[21] reports that asthma did not affect the outcome after ESS when comparing patients with equally severe sinus disease, except for the worst patients, in whom asthma did adversely affect the outcome.

Until recently, no well-conducted clinical trials have been performed showing beneficial effects of medical therapy for CRS on bronchial asthma. Ragab and colleagues[22] published the first prospective study of surgical compared with medical therapy for 43 patients with CRS with or without NP and asthma. Medical therapy consisted of a 12-week course of erythromycin, alkaline nasal douches, and intranasal corticosteroid preparation, followed by intranasal corticosteroid preparation tailored to the patients' clinical course. The surgical treatment group underwent ESS followed by a 2-week course of erythromycin, alkaline nasal douches, and intranasal corticosteroid preparation, 3 months of alkaline nasal douches and intranasal corticosteroid, followed by intranasal corticosteroid preparation tailored to the patients' clinical course. Both medical as well as surgical treatment regimens for CRS were associated with subjective and objective improvements in asthma state. Of note, improvement in upper airway symptoms correlated with improvement in asthma symptoms and control.

RHINOSINUSITIS WITH NASAL POLYPS AND ASTHMA
Prevalence

Seven percent of asthma patients have NP.[1] In nonatopic asthma and late-onset asthma, polyps are diagnosed more frequently (10%–15%). Aspirin-induced asthma is a distinct clinical syndrome characterized by the triad aspirin sensitivity, asthma, and nasal polyposis, and has an estimated prevalence of 1% in the general population and 10% among asthmatics.[1]

Pathophysiology

At present, the etiology of NP remains obscure.[3] As nasal polyps represent a chronic inflammatory disease affecting the mucosa of ethmoidal sinus cavities in susceptible individuals, one may speculate on airborne microorganisms being able to induce or aggravate the inflammation seen in NP. New light was recently shed on the pathology of NP by a report showing increased colonization of NP by *S. aureus* and presence of specific IgE directed against *S. aureus* enterotoxins in NP tissue.[23] Of note, rates of colonization and IgE presence in NP tissue were increased in subjects with NP and comorbid asthma or aspirin sensitivity. By their superantigenic activity, enterotoxins may activate inflammatory cells in an antigen-unspecific way. Hellings and colleagues[17] recently demonstrated that nasal application of *S. aureus* enterotoxin B is capable of aggravating experimental allergic rhinitis and asthma, with an increase in bronchial and systemic Th2 cytokine levels. Besides bacterial enterotoxins, Ponikau and colleagues[24] report on the potentially important role of fungi, especially *Alternaria*, in the generation of NP. By their capacity to induce eosinophil degranulation, *Alternaria* may contribute to the inflammatory spectrum of CRS with or without NP. To date it is unknown whether microbial stimuli may represent the etiology of NP formation or whether colonization with microorganisms is favored in the presence of NP.

Treatment

At present, no trials have been performed studying the effects of medical therapy for NP patients on asthma. Therefore, well-designed trials on antibiotic use, vaccination therapy, or antileukotriene treatment in patients with NP and asthma are warranted. After ESS for NP in patients with concomitant asthma, a significant improvement in lung function and a reduction of systemic steroid use was noted, whereas this was not the case in aspirin-intolerant asthma patients.[25]

RHINOSINUSITIS AND CHRONIC OBSTRUCTIVE PULMONARY DISEASE

Up to 88% of patients with COPD presenting at an academic unit of respiratory disease may experience nasal symptoms, most commonly rhinorrhea.[2] Nasal symptoms in COPD patients correspond well with an overall impairment of the quality of life. So far, there is only one study in patients with COPD showing rhinosinusitis symptoms and inflammatory mediators in the nasal cavity.[2] Of note, patients with stable COPD show increased levels of eotaxin and G-CSF in nasal lavage fluid compared with controls.[2] It remains to be elucidated to what extent treatment of the nose is beneficial in COPD.

CLINICAL IMPLICATIONS AND UNMET NEEDS

Several medical specialties are involved in the medical care of patients with chronic airway disease. In asthmatic and COPD patients, physicians need to inquire routinely about the existence of upper airway symptoms. To this purpose, the use of a simple questionnaire for the presence of sinonasal symptoms may be helpful to the clinician. In the case of positive history for upper airway symptoms, anterior rhinoscopy, nasal endoscopy, or computed tomography scan of the sinonasal cavity can help in making a correct estimation of upper airway involvement in asthma and COPD. Alternatively, bronchial symptoms need to be asked for in patients presenting with rhinitis and rhinosinusitis. When lung function tests are performed in this patient population, most of them will show bronchial hyperresponsiveness, making the clinician aware of the global airway impact of the upper airway disease. However, several clues to fully understand the nasobronchial interaction are still missing, complicating the clinical approach toward individuals with upper or lower airway disease. For example, one cannot predict in individual patients with rhinitis if and when rhinitis will progress to the development of bronchial symptoms. It may therefore be important to evaluate bronchial function in all patients with persistent rhinitis symptoms. In patients with NP and concomitant asthma or COPD, it is not known whether sinus surgery or any other medical treatment of rhinosinusitis will have beneficial effects on lower airway pathology. Therefore, prospective clinical trials on outcomes of upper airway therapy should not only concentrate on parameters of upper airway disease but also take into account the effects of treatment on lower airways. Alternatively, the impact of asthma or COPD on rhinosinusitis remains obscure. As upper airway inflammation may be induced by bronchial inflammation,[26] rhinologists need to closely collaborate with pneumologists to design a therapeutic strategy aimed at obtaining the optimal condition for both parts of the airway.

A minority of CRS and asthma patients are refractory to standard medical therapy and sinus surgery procedures. In these patients, the disease development still remains incompletely understood. Therefore, one of the future tasks that remains is to delineate factors that contribute to severe CRS and asthma-like exposure to environmental or occupational agents, underlying gastroesophageal reflux, or infection or colonization with microorganisms. Fungal extracts and bacterial enterotoxins have been linked recently to the etiology of NP. Research in microbial triggers and their interplay with airway biology should be extended to viruses and atypical bacteria such as *Mycoplasma* and *Chlamydia*. In addition, the cellular source and the mechanisms of systemic release of proinflammatory mediators, such as IL-5 and eotaxin, by allergen inhalation are still unknown. Whether the systemic release of these mediators represents diffusion of locally produced molecules, or rather systemic release by circulating cells, remains to be explored. After full comprehension of the mechanisms of systemic mediator release, novel treatment strategies can be designed, aimed at reducing the systemic immune response with its impact on global airway disease.

For clinical practice, there is a need for noninvasive markers of inflammation in upper and lower airways. Among noninvasive biologic markers of inflammation, nasal and bronchial nitric oxide (NO) measurement may represent a novel tool for diagnostic purposes as well as for the prediction of the success of therapy. Despite the validity of NO measurements in exhaled air in asthma patients,[27] its role in upper airway inflammation needs to be studied further. Induced sputum, another noninvasive tool for research, may provide relevant information on the involvement of bronchial inflammation in patients with upper airway disease. Further studies are needed for delineating its validity in rhinologic practice.

SUMMARY

Upper and lower airway inflammation share common pathophysiologic pathways, frequently coexist, and communicate via the systemic circulation. The threshold for developing symptoms in upper and lower airways relates to intrinsic and extrinsic factors. Genetic predisposition, organ susceptibility, and breathing patterns are likely to be involved in the development of bronchial symptoms in patients with rhinosinusitis. Extrinsic factors such as the dose of exposed allergens in atopic patients, the microbial environment, and occupational factors may all contribute to the complex picture of global airway disease. Many unanswered questions relate to the generation of symptoms in patients with airway inflammation. However, the awareness of bronchial symptoms in patients with upper airway inflammation, and vice versa, may at this stage represent a major step forward in the diagnostic and therapeutic approach. The full appreciation of involvement of upper and lower airway disease in one patient can only be executed in a multidisciplinary clinical setting, involving doctors being able to examine and interpret clinical abnormalities of upper and lower airways. Anterior rhinoscopy and nasal endoscopy should be combined with lung function tests in patients with any chronic airway disorder. The validation of noninvasive parameters of airway inflammation such as NO measurement, and the optimization of combined treatment strategies for patients with upper or lower airway disease, will be major tasks for the upcoming decade.

REFERENCES

1. Hens G, Hellings PW. The nose: gatekeeper and trigger of bronchial disease. Rhinology 2006;44:179–87.
2. Hens G, Vanaudenaerde BM, Bullens DM, et al. Sinonasal pathology in nonallergic asthma and COPD: 'united airway disease' beyond the scope of allergy. Allergy 2008;63:261–7.
3. Fokkens W, Lund V, Mullol J. European position paper on rhinosinusitis and nasal polyps 2007. Rhinol Suppl 2007;20:1–136.
4. Denburg JA, Keith PK. Systemic aspects of chronic rhinosinusitis. Immunol Allergy Clin North Am 2004;24:87–102.
5. Turner RB. Epidemiology, pathogenesis, and treatment of the common cold. Ann Allergy Asthma Immunol 1997;78:531–9 [quiz 539–40].
6. Johnston SL, Pattemore PK, Sanderson G, et al. Community study of role of viral infections in exacerbations of asthma in 9–11 year old children. BMJ 1995;310:1225–9.
7. Grunberg K, Timmers MC, de Klerk EP, et al. Experimental rhinovirus 16 infection causes variable airway obstruction in subjects with atopic asthma. Am J Respir Crit Care Med 1999;160:1375–80.
8. Lemanske RF Jr, Dick EC, Swenson CA, et al. Rhinovirus upper respiratory infection increases airway hyperreactivity and late asthmatic reactions. J Clin Invest 1989;83:1–10.
9. Seemungal T, Harper-Owen R, Bhowmik A, et al. Respiratory viruses, symptoms, and inflammatory markers in acute exacerbations and stable chronic obstructive pulmonary disease. Am J Respir Crit Care Med 2001;164:1618–23.
10. Papadopoulos NG, Bates PJ, Bardin PG, et al. Rhinoviruses infect the lower airways. J Infect Dis 2000;181:1875–84.
11. Mosser AG, Vrtis R, Burchell L, et al. Quantitative and qualitative analysis of rhinovirus infection in bronchial tissues. Am J Respir Crit Care Med 2005;171:645–51.

12. Gern JE. Rhinovirus respiratory infections and asthma. Am J Med 2002; 112(Suppl 6A):19S–27S.
13. Avila PC, Abisheganaden JA, Wong H, et al. Effects of allergic inflammation of the nasal mucosa on the severity of rhinovirus 16 cold. J Allergy Clin Immunol 2000; 105:923–32.
14. Edwards MR, Kebadze T, Johnson MW, et al. New treatment regimes for virus-induced exacerbations of asthma. Pulm Pharmacol Ther 2006;19:320–34.
15. Ponikau JU, Sherris DA, Kephart GM, et al. Features of airway remodeling and eosinophilic inflammation in chronic rhinosinusitis: is the histopathology similar to asthma? J Allergy Clin Immunol 2003;112:877–82.
16. Ragab A, Clement P, Vincken W. Correlation between the cytology of the nasal middle meatus and BAL in chronic rhinosinusitis. Rhinology 2005;43:11–7.
17. Hellings PW, Hens G, Meyts I, et al. Aggravation of bronchial eosinophilia in mice by nasal and bronchial exposure to *Staphylococcus aureus* enterotoxin B. Clin Exp Allergy 2006;36:1063–71.
18. Senior BA, Kennedy DW, Tanabodee J, et al. Long-term impact of functional endoscopic sinus surgery on asthma. Otolaryngol Head Neck Surg 1999;121: 66–8.
19. Manning SC, Wasserman RL, Silver R, et al. Results of endoscopic sinus surgery in pediatric patients with chronic sinusitis and asthma. Arch Otolaryngol Head Neck Surg 1994;120:1142–5.
20. Schaitkin B, May M, Shapiro A, et al. Endoscopic sinus surgery: 4-year follow-up on the first 100 patients. Laryngoscope 1993;103:1117–20.
21. Kennedy DW. Prognostic factors, outcomes and staging in ethmoid sinus surgery. Laryngoscope 1992;102:1–18.
22. Ragab S, Scadding GK, Lund VJ, et al. Treatment of chronic rhinosinusitis and its effects on asthma. Eur Respir J 2006;28:68–74.
23. Van Zele T, Gevaert P, Watelet JB, et al. *Staphylococcus aureus* colonization and IgE antibody formation to enterotoxins is increased in nasal polyposis. J Allergy Clin Immunol 2004;114:981–3.
24. Ponikau JU, Sherris DA, Kephart GM, et al. The role of ubiquitous airborne fungi in chronic rhinosinusitis. Curr Allergy Asthma Rep 2005;5:472–6.
25. Batra PS, Kern RC, Tripathi A, et al. Outcome analysis of endoscopic sinus surgery in patients with nasal polyps and asthma. Laryngoscope 2003;113: 1703–6.
26. Braunstahl GJ, Hellings PW. Nasobronchial interaction mechanisms in allergic airways disease. Curr Opin Otolaryngol Head Neck Surg 2006;14:176–82.
27. Scadding G. Nitric oxide in the airways. Curr Opin Otolaryngol Head Neck Surg 2007;15:258–63.

Index

Note: Page numbers of article titles are in **boldface** type.

A

United States Postal Service

Statement of Ownership, Management, and Circulation
(All Periodicals Publications Except Requestor Publications)

1. Publication Title
Immunology and Allergy Clinics of North America

2. Publication Number
0 0 6 - 3 6 1

3. Filing Date
9/15/09

4. Issue Frequency
Feb, May, Aug, Nov

5. Number of Issues Published Annually
4

6. Annual Subscription Price
$233.00

7. Complete Mailing Address of Known Office of Publication (Not printer) (Street, city, county, state, and ZIP+4®)

Elsevier Inc.
360 Park Avenue South
New York, NY 10010-1710

Contact Person
Stephen Bushing

Telephone (Include area code)
215-239-3688

8. Complete Mailing Address of Headquarters or General Business Office of Publisher (Not printer)
Elsevier Inc., 360 Park Avenue South, New York, NY 10010-1710

9. Full Names and Complete Mailing Addresses of Publisher, Editor, and Managing Editor (Do not leave blank)

Publisher (Name and complete mailing address)
John Schrefer, Elsevier, Inc., 1600 John F. Kennedy Blvd. Suite 1800, Philadelphia, PA 19103-2899

Editor (Name and complete mailing address)
Patrick Manley, Elsevier, Inc., 1600 John F. Kennedy Blvd. Suite 1800, Philadelphia, PA 19103-2899

Managing Editor (Name and complete mailing address)
Catherine Bewick, Elsevier, Inc., 1600 John F. Kennedy Blvd. Suite 1800, Philadelphia, PA 19103-2899

10. Owner (Do not leave blank. If the publication is owned by a corporation, give the name and address of the corporation immediately followed by the names and addresses of all stockholders owning or holding 1 percent or more of the total amount of stock. If not owned by a corporation, give the names and addresses of the individual owners. If owned by a partnership or other unincorporated firm, give its name and address as well as those of each individual owner. If the publication is published by a nonprofit organization, give its name and address.)

Full Name	Complete Mailing Address
Wholly owned subsidiary of	4520 East-West Highway
Reed/Elsevier, US holdings	Bethesda, MD 20814

11. Known Bondholders, Mortgagees, and Other Security Holders Owning or Holding 1 Percent or More of Total Amount of Bonds, Mortgages, or Other Securities. If none, check box ☑ None

Full Name	Complete Mailing Address
N/A	

12. Tax Status (For completion by nonprofit organizations authorized to mail at nonprofit rates) (Check one)
The purpose, function, and nonprofit status of this organization and the exempt status for federal income tax purposes:
☐ Has Not Changed During Preceding 12 Months
☐ Has Changed During Preceding 12 Months (Publisher must submit explanation of change with this statement)

PS Form 3526, September 2007 (Page 1 of 3) (Instructions Page 3)) PSN 7530-01-000-9931 PRIVACY NOTICE. See our Privacy policy in www.usps.com

---

13. Publication Title
Immunology and Allergy Clinics of North America

14. Issue Date for Circulation Data Below
August 2009

15. Extent and Nature of Circulation			Average No. Copies Each Issue During Preceding 12 Months	No. Copies of Single Issue Published Nearest to Filing Date
a. Total Number of Copies (Net press run)			1200	1200
b. Paid Circulation (By Mail and Outside the Mail)	(1)	Mailed Outside-County Paid Subscriptions Stated on PS Form 3541 (Include paid distribution above nominal rate, advertiser's proof copies, and exchange copies)	482	478
	(2)	Mailed In-County Paid Subscriptions Stated on PS Form 3541 (Include paid distribution above nominal rate, advertiser's proof copies, and exchange copies)		
	(3)	Paid Distribution Outside the Mails Including Sales Through Dealers and Carriers, Street Vendors, Counter Sales, and Other Paid Distribution Outside USPS®	137	133
	(4)	Paid Distribution by Other Classes Mailed Through the USPS (e.g. First-Class Mail®)		
c. Total Paid Distribution (Sum of 15b (1), (2), (3), and (4))		▲	619	611
d. Free or Nominal Rate Distribution (By Mail and Outside the Mail)	(1)	Free or Nominal Rate Outside-County Copies Included on PS Form 3541	72	79
	(2)	Free or Nominal Rate In-County Copies Included on PS Form 3541		
	(3)	Free or Nominal Rate Copies Mailed at Other Classes Through the USPS (e.g. First-Class Mail)		
	(4)	Free or Nominal Rate Distribution Outside the Mail (Carriers or other means)		
e. Total Free or Nominal Rate Distribution (Sum of 15d (1), (2), (3) and (4))		▲	72	79
f. Total Distribution (Sum of 15c and 15e)		▲	691	690
g. Copies not Distributed (See instructions to publishers #4 (page #3))		▲	509	510
h. Total (Sum of 15f and g)			1200	1200
i. Percent Paid (15c divided by 15f times 100)			89.58%	88.55%

16. Publication of Statement of Ownership

If the publication is a general publication, publication of this statement is required. Will be printed ☑ Publication not required
in the **November 2009** issue of this publication.

17. Signature and Title of Editor, Publisher, Business Manager, or Owner

Stephen R. Bushing

Stephen R. Bushing – Subscription Services Coordinator

Date September 15, 2009

I certify that all information furnished on this form is true and complete. I understand that anyone who furnishes false or misleading information on this form or who omits material or information requested on the form may be subject to criminal sanctions (including fines and imprisonment) and/or civil sanctions (including civil penalties).

PS Form 3526, September 2007 (Page 2 of 3)

Moving?

Make sure your subscription moves with you!

To notify us of your new address, find your **Clinics Account Number** (located on your mailing label above your name), and contact customer service at:

Email: journalscustomerservice-usa@elsevier.com

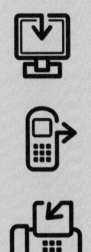

800-654-2452 (subscribers in the U.S. & Canada)
314-447-8871 (subscribers outside of the U.S. & Canada)

Fax number: 314-447-8029

Elsevier Health Sciences Division
Subscription Customer Service
3251 Riverport Lane
Maryland Heights, MO 63043

*To ensure uninterrupted delivery of your subscription, please notify us at least 4 weeks in advance of move.

Printed and bound by CPI Group (UK) Ltd, Croydon, CR0 4YY

03/10/2024

01040464-0007